A PSYCHIATRIC
VADE-MECUM

by

Basant K Puri MA, MB, BChir, MRCPsych

Consultant Psychiatrist and Honorary Senior Lecturer,
Imperial College School of Medicine,
Hammersmith Hospital,
London, UK

and

Heather McKee MB, BCh, MRCPsych

Consultant Psychiatrist,
Charing Cross Hospital,
London, UK

A member of the Hodder Headline Group
LONDON · SYDNEY · AUCKLAND
Co-published in the United States of America by
Oxford University Press Inc., New York

6

First published in Great Britain in 1998 by
Arnold, a member of the Hodder Headline Group,
338 Euston Road, London NW1 3BH

http://www.arnoldpublishers.com

Co-published in the United States of America by
Oxford University Press Inc.,
198 Madison Avenue, New York, NY 10016
Oxford is a registered trademark of Oxford University Press

Whilst the advice and information in this book is believed to be true and
accurate at the date of going to press, neither the authors nor the publisher
can accept any legal responsibility or liability for any errors or omissions
that may be made. In particular (but without limiting the generality of the
preceding disclaimer) every effort has been made to check drug dosages;
however, it is still possible that errors have been missed. Furthermore,
dosage schedules are constantly being revised and new side-effects
recognized. For these reasons the reader is strongly urged to consult the
drug companies' printed instructions before administering any of the drugs
recommended in this book.

British Library Cataloguing in Publication Data
A catalogue record for this book is available from the British Library

Library of Congress Cataloging-in-Publication Data
A catalog record for this book is available from the Library of Congress

ISBN 0 340 69171 9

1 2 3 4 5 6 7 8 9 10

Commissioning Editor: Georgina Bentliff
Production Editor: Wendy Rooke
Production Controller: Rose James
Cover Design: Terry Griffiths

Typeset in 8/10pt New Baskerville by
Photoprint Typesetting, Torquay, Devon
Printed and bound in Hong Kong by
Colorcraft Ltd

CONTENTS

PREFACE

This pocket-book is written primarily for psychiatric and general practice trainees, and is designed to be used when they are on call or going about their daily work. It deals with topics involved in the admission and assessment of a psychiatric patient and goes on to cover diagnosis, treatment, discharge and aspects of community care, as well as some essential medico-legal topics. The book also provides some practical guidance for trainee doctors, for example regarding their career, their tutor's role, and dealing with stress.

Basant Puri
Heather McKee
1998

Part I

Admission
and
Assessment

1

GOOD MEDICAL PRACTICE

The General Medical Council (GMC) published, in October 1995, *The Duties of a Doctor*. This consists of the following four booklets which provide advice on the standards of practice and care that the GMC believes patients have a right to expect of doctors.

- *Good Medical Practice* – the core booklet of guidance setting out the standards which the GMC expects all doctors to meet when working with patients and colleagues, in their clinical practice and other professional roles.
- *Confidentiality.*
- *Advertising.*
- *HIV Infection and AIDS.*

According to *Good Medical Practice*, patients must be able to trust doctors with their lives and well-being. To justify that trust, we as a profession have a duty to maintain a good standard of practice and care, and to show respect for human life. As a doctor, you must:

- make the care of your patient your first concern;
- treat every patient politely and considerately;
- respect patients' dignity and privacy;
- listen to patients and respect their views;
- give patients information in a form that they can understand;
- respect the rights of patients to be fully involved in decisions about their care;
- keep your professional knowledge and skills up to date;

- recognize the limits of your professional competence;
- be honest and trustworthy;
- respect and protect confidential information;
- make sure that your personal beliefs do not prejudice your patients' care;
- act quickly to protect patients from a risk if you have good reason to believe that you or a colleague may not be fit to practise;
- avoid abusing your position as a doctor;
- work with colleagues in the ways that best serve patients' interests.

PROFESSIONAL RELATIONSHIPS WITH PATIENTS

The following additional guidance has been given by the General Medical Council (GMC) in *The Duties of a Doctor* (October 1995):

Successful relationships between doctors and patients depend on trust.

To establish and maintain that trust you must:

- give patients the information they ask for or need about their condition, its treatment and prognosis;
- respect the right of patients to refuse treatment or take part in teaching or research;
- respect the right of patients to a second opinion;
- ask patients' permission, if possible, before sharing information with their spouses, partners or relatives;
- be accessible to patients when you are on duty;
- respond to criticisms and complaints promptly and constructively.

You must not allow your views about a patient's lifestyle, culture, beliefs, race, colour, sex, sexuality, age, social status or perceived economic worth to prejudice the treatment you give or arrange.

If you feel that your beliefs might affect the treatment you provide, you must explain this to patients, and inform them of their right to see another doctor.

You must not refuse or delay treatment because you believe that a patient's actions have contributed

5

to his or her condition, or because you may be putting yourself at risk.

Because the doctor–patient relationship is based on trust, you have a special responsibility to make the relationship with your patients work. If the trust between you and a patient breaks down, either of you may end the relationship. If this happens, you must do your best to make sure that arrangements are made promptly for the continuing care of the patient. You should hand over records or other information for use by the new doctor as soon as possible.

3

THE ROLE OF THE JUNIOR DOCTOR (INCLUDING LINES OF RESPONSIBILITY)

Junior doctors working in psychiatry can be taking part in a 3-year organized training scheme with a view to taking Membership examinations of the Royal College of Psychiatrists. Alternatively, they may be training to become members of the Royal College of General Practitioners or, more rarely, they may be spending a short period in psychiatry in order to gain further experience as part of an alternative career pathway.

A junior doctor is usually attached to a 'firm' and has a trainer who is a consultant as well as a psychiatric tutor. The 'firm' may also have a senior registrar or staff-grade doctor who will work as part of a team with the junior doctor.

The trainer supervises the junior doctor both formally and informally. The formal supervision consists of an hour a week when progress can be assessed. Informal supervision takes place at out-patient clinics and ward rounds and also as other opportunities arise.

The junior doctor learns about psychiatry partly within an 'apprenticeship' model, but should also take part in afternoon release teaching sessions and academic afternoons at the hospital where he or she works, including journal clubs, case presentations and lectures by visiting lecturers.

The work of the junior doctor depends on the environment in which he or she is working, but the most common situation is to work in a ward or day hospital where the doctor is responsible for the day-to-day care of the patients, along with the other members of the multidisciplinary team.

Patients are interviewed, notes are taken and daily problems and variations are dealt with.

Care plans are written initially and updated at ward rounds, and medication cards are usually the remit of the junior doctor, but all doctors in the team can feel free to rewrite the medicine charts when required.

Discharged summaries are written promptly by the junior doctor, who liaises with the general practitioner. Any patients who require medical opinions will usually have this attended to by the junior doctor.

The junior doctor has a key role, and he or she usually establishes rapport with the patients and other members of the multidisciplinary teams such as nurses, occupational therapists and psychologists.

The relationship with the trainer, the consultant, is essentially that of a role model and lays a foundation of knowledge on dealing with difficult situations. At any time when a problem arises the junior doctor is able to ask the consultant or senior registrar for advice, and the work of the junior doctor is monitored. Should there be a problem of a personal nature at any time, such as relationship or examination difficulties, the 'pastoral' role of the trainer is there if the junior doctor wishes to avail him- or herself of it. Should the trainer and the trainee not have an adequate rapport to enable them to deal with problems the psychiatric tutor is usually well attuned to these particular types of problems and can be approached instead. The trainer and other members of the team can arrange 'mock examinations' and suggest studying techniques when examinations loom, as well as encouraging anxious candidates and building their confidence.

Junior doctors are on the 'on-call' rota, which means that they stay in the hospital over 24 hours or 12 hours, depending on the stipulations of their rota, and see any new referrals over that period. This responsibility can be quite onerous and sometimes stressful. The ability to cope with 'on-call' depends on the doctor, the amount of work, and the support received by the doctor.

There is always a consultant 'on call' and sometimes, depending on how busy the job is, there may be a senior registrar as well. Junior doctors can be quite reluctant to ask for help, and sometimes consultants may be equally reluctant to offer it, but it is not a sign of weakness to know your limitations, and it is the 'on-call' consultant's ultimate responsibility. The 'on-call' aspect of the junior doctor's work can be difficult to support and supervise and various methods are adopted. These consist of writing down the details of all the patients seen and the interventions and discussing these with the 'on-call' consultant the next day. Sometimes the junior doctor will telephone the consultant or the consultant will telephone the junior doctor during the 'on-call' period.

Inevitably the junior doctor will have a greater degree of autonomy 'on call' than he or she perhaps has at any other time. Junior doctors require an adequate induction and induction literature when they initially are 'on call', which may be the first night that they start to work in that area without knowing either the catchment areas or the degree of specialism required.

4

THE ROLE OF THE RESPONSIBLE MEDICAL OFFICER (RMO)

The responsible medical officer (RMO) will usually be a consultant psychiatrist on the staff of a hospital (NHS or private) to which the patient has been admitted. This applies to individuals detained for assessment or treatment under the Mental Health Act 1983, or who are subject to aftercare under supervision after being discharged. The RMO does not have to be approved under Section 12, but this will almost always be the case.

When the consultant is absent due to annual leave or sickness, the doctor in charge of the patient's treatment will act as the RMO. This person should be a consultant, but may not always be so.

Although the RMO has a leading role in the clinical team treating the patient, he or she does not have overall management accountability for the treatment that the patient receives from others.

The RMO is involved in the following.

Reclassification of patients
When a patient who has been detained appears to the RMO to be suffering from a different mental disorder to that on the application, he or she will provide the managers with a report to this effect so that the application with the new mental disorder can be implemented. Similarly, in the event of psychopathic disorder and mental impairment the RMO should also provide a report that includes the issue of treatment response, and if treatment is

unlikely to influence the outcome, the managers will cease to detain the patient.

Renewal of detention

Patients who are detained for treatment or placed under guardianship are examined by the RMO 2 months before they cease to be liable to be detained, and a decision is made as to whether they may be suffering from mental illness, severe mental impairment, psychopathic disorder or mental impairment and if treatment is going to alleviate or prevent deterioration of the condition. A decision as to what is necessary for the health and safety of the patient or for the protection of others needs to be made.

The RMO should consult the people involved professionally with the patient's medical treatment and provide a report to the managers if he or she feels that a renewal of the treatment (guardianship) order is necessary.

Leave of absence from hospital

The RMO may grant to any detained patient (except those detained under the authority of the Home Secretary) leave of absence from the hospital. This may be accompanied or unaccompanied, and must state the conditions which the medical officer feels are necessary both for the interests of the patient and for the safety of others. For example, a patient who is concerned about the safety of his or her home could go there accompanied by a nurse for reassurance, or for unaccompanied weekend leave in order to gain confidence after a period of hospitalization.

The leave conditions should be recorded appropriately on a Section 17 leave form. Only the RMO can grant leave.

Consent to treatment

Medical treatment for the purposes of the Mental Health Act 1983 includes 'nursing and care, habilitation and rehabilitation under medical supervision'. It includes physical treatments such as electroconvulsive therapy (ECT), psychotropic drug administration and psychotherapy. The old Mental Health Act 1959 implied that compulsory detention in hospital gave an automatic right to the doctor to treat the problem from which the patient suffered.

Parliament has now decided that fulfilling the criteria for compulsory detention does not mean that the patient is always incompetent. Patients can sometimes give informed consent to treatment, and should always be given the opportunity to understand the purpose of the treatment and agree to it or refuse accordingly.

However, the RMO may decide, usually with the consensus of the multidisciplinary team, that the patient should have the treatment even if he or she refuses or is unable to refuse because of his or her mental disorder.

Part IV of the Mental Health Act 1983 lays out the procedures needed in law for the RMO to give certain treatments to detained refusing patients and, in certain cases, other treatments:

- treatments requiring consent *and* a second opinion – Section 57;
- treatments requiring consent *or* a second opinion – Section 58;
- treatments not requiring consent – Section 63.

Treatments requiring consent and *a second opinion* – *Section 57*

These include the following:

1. psychosurgery;
2. surgical implantation of hormones to reduce male sexual drive, but:
   - the patient must give his informed consent;
   - an independent doctor and two non-medical persons from the Mental Health Act Commission must state that the patient is capable of giving informed consent;

- the independent doctor, after talking to staff, must certify that the treatment will alleviate or prevent further deterioration in the patient's condition.

Treatments requiring consent or *a second opinion –*
Section 58

These include the following:

1. ECT;
2. the administration of medicine to a detained patient 3 months after medicine has first been given by any means.

A patient shall not be given any treatment to which Section 58 applies unless:

- the patient has consented to the treatment and either the RMO or an appropriate doctor has certified in writing that the patient is capable of giving informed consent;
- an appointed doctor has certified in writing that the patient is not capable of giving informed consent but, because the treatment is likely to alleviate or prevent further deterioration, the appointed doctor certifies that it should be given;
- the patient has refused consent, and may or may not be capable of giving informed consent, but the appointed doctor certifies in writing that treatment should be given as it is likely to improve the patient's mental condition or prevent further deterioration. Drugs prescribed solely for the treatment of physical illness do not fall within the scope of the Act.

If patients do not consent to appropriate treatment, an opinion is sought from a second opinion appointed doctor (SOAD) who is appointed by the Mental Health Act Commission, and whose role is to give his or her opinion on consent and treatment. He or she reviews the patient's ability to give consent and the treatment plan, and talks to a nurse and a non-nursing member of staff involved in the treatment of the patient. The appointed doctor will usually expect to discuss the treatment with the RMO and agree a treatment plan. It is expected that the SOAD will support a consultant proposing a treatment that others would regard as the expected mode of treatment. Occasionally, if either doctor is idiosyncratic in his or her treatment plans, this will not work, and the Act does not provide for a formal appeals procedure. However, should the patient's circumstances change, the RMO should contact the Regional Commission office who will again refer the case to the appointed doctor, who will usually visit to consider the new situation.

Urgent treatment (Section 62)
Treatments which would otherwise require consent and/or a second opinion may be given by the RMO in urgent situations:

- to save the patient's life (e.g. if he or she is not eating or drinking);
- in a situation where it is immediately necessary to prevent serious suffering by the patient;
- in a situation where it is immediately necessary and minimum interference is needed to prevent the patient from being violent or becoming a danger to himself, herself or others.

In cases where a treatment (e.g. an urgent surgical operation) needs to be given for a physical disorder to a patient who is unable to provide informed consent, such that the treatment does not come within the scope of the Mental Health Act, then this treatment will be governed by common law and the Mental Health Act Commission does not have a role.

CONSENT TO TREATMENT AND INVESTIGATION

In June 1993 the GMC published the following statement on consent to investigation or treatment:

It has long been accepted, and is well understood within the profession, that a doctor should treat a patient only on the basis of the patient's informed consent. Doctors are expected in all normal circumstances to be sure that their patients consent to the carrying out of investigative procedures involving the removal of samples or invasive techniques, whether those investigations are performed for the purposes of routine screening, for example in pregnancy or prior to surgery, or for the more specific purpose of differential diagnosis. A patient's consent may in certain circumstances be given implicitly, for example by agreement to provide a specimen of blood for multiple analysis. In other circumstances it needs to be given explicitly, for example before undergoing a specified operative procedure or providing a specimen of blood to be tested specifically for a named condition. As the expectations of patients, and consequently the demands made upon doctors, increase and develop, it is essential that both doctor and patient feel free to exchange information before investigation or treatment is undertaken.

Thus the doctor has a duty to discuss the benefits and risks of a treatment with the patient, and to obtain consent for that treatment. Treatment may be administered without consent if the patient is detained under an appropriate Section of the Mental Health Act (MHA) allowing such treatment. In particular, in the case of an *informal* patient, treatment must never be enforced without consent *if there is time* to implement an appropriate emergency section of the MHA; such a course of action could be construed as constituting assault. Note that, none the less, emergency Sections do not allow compulsory treatment of patients. However, remember that in emergency situations relating to an informal patient in which there is not sufficient time to invoke an emergency Section, *under common law* a doctor has the duty to preserve life and to prevent serious injury to the patient or others.

ADMITTING PSYCHIATRIC PATIENTS

HOSPITALIZATION

Most patients with psychiatric disorders can be assessed and managed as out-patients. However, there are cases when hospitalization is necessary, such as when:

- the patient's life is at risk from suicidal thoughts, e.g. in depression and schizophrenia;
- a dangerous level of self-neglect is likely, e.g. in mania;
- severe weight loss and electrolyte loss have occurred, e.g. in anorexia nervosa;
- appropriate investigations need to be carried out, e.g. first-episode schizophrenia/schizophreniform disorder;
- the patient represents a danger to others.

Patients recovering from a psychiatric disorder who require some help during the day, but not full in-patient care, may be admitted to a day hospital which they attend on an agreed number of days each week; their mental state and response to medication can be monitored, and they may be offered therapeutic activities, e.g. occupational therapy.

INFORMAL ADMISSIONS

Most admissions to psychiatric in-patient units are informal, i.e. voluntary.

COMPULSORY (FORMAL) ADMISSIONS

When a patient with a psychiatric disorder requires hospitalization but cannot be admitted informally, a formal or compulsory admission is necessary, under the appropriate mental health legislation as follows:

- in England and Wales – the *Mental Health Act 1983* and *The Code of Practice – Mental Health Act 1983*;
- in Scotland – the *Mental Health (Scotland) Act 1984*;
- in Northern Ireland – *the Mental Health (Northern Ireland) Order 1986.*

According to *The Health of the Nation*:

Detention of a person in hospital, either for assessment or treatment, is properly and entirely a matter for the professional judgement of the doctors and social workers concerned and people may only be compulsorily detained if the criteria laid down in the Mental Health Act 1983 are met. Under the Act an individual who is mentally disordered may be admitted compulsorily to hospital where this is necessary:

- in the interests of his or her own health; *or*
- in the interests of his or her own safety; *or*
- for the protection of other people.

Only one of the above grounds needs to be satisfied.

PROCEDURE

Once it is clear that a patient requires admission for psychiatric assessment and/or treatment, the GP should first try to persuade the patient to be admitted informally. If the patient does not protest against this, the informal admission may then be organized in the usual way by contacting the duty psychiatrist.

If the patient refuses informal admission, then he or she will need to be assessed for compulsory admission. The following account is written primarily with the Mental Health Act 1983 (England and Wales) (MHA) in mind, but other mental health legislation is often similar, particularly in Scotland,

Northern Ireland and Eire. (Definitions of particular terms, such as Approved Social Worker, and a summary of the main Sections are given in the penultimate section of this book, under Mental Health Legislation.)

The GP should contact the Approved Social Worker. It is the Approved Social Worker who applies for compulsory admission under the MHA. The local hospital switchboard, police station or social services department will have details of the on-call Approved Social Worker. Although under the MHA the nearest relative can be the applicant, the *Code of Practice* makes it clear that the Approved Social Worker is usually the right applicant. In most circumstances the doctor should therefore advise the nearest relative that it is preferable for the Approved Social Worker to make an assessment of the need for the patient to be admitted under the MHA. If necessary, for example because the Approved Social Worker cannot be contacted, the nearest relative can be advised of his or her right to make an application. However, the nearest relative should never be advised to make the application simply in order to avoid involving an Approved Social Worker in the assessment.

For a patient in the community, the Approved Social Worker will normally contact an Approved Doctor, carry the relevant forms and generally coordinate the assessment. In the case of a patient already in hospital the Senior House Officer (SHO) of the clinical team in charge of the case will fulfil this role.

Prior to the assessment it is important for the GP to gather as much relevant information as possible about the patient. In the case of a patient in the community, this may be carried out by consulting colleagues in the same practice, and discussing the case with the patient's relatives and the local psychiatric unit. Particular attention should be paid to evidence relating to the health and/or safety of the patient, the risk of harm to others, and unusual behaviour which may be indicative of the presence of mental disorder. The mental health assessment should be arranged in such a way that the participants are able to meet, for example outside the patient's home, for a preliminary discussion regarding the conduct of the assessment. In the case of a patient who is already in hospital, it is important for the GP to discuss the case with members of the medical and nursing staff and to peruse the case-notes.

According to the *Code of Practice* a proper medical examination requires:

- direct personal examination of the patient's mental state, taking into account the social, cultural and (where relevant) ethnic context;
- consideration of all available relevant medical information, including that in the possession of others, be they professional or non-professional.

Once the patient has been examined and the relevant forms filled in, the application should be addressed to the hospital managers.

SPECIAL CONSIDERATIONS

If the patient and doctor cannot understand each other's language the doctor should, wherever practicable, have recourse to a professional interpreter, including a professional signer in the case of a patient with hearing difficulties who understands sign language; the interpreter or signer should understand the terminology and conduct of psychiatric interviews.

'DIFFICULT' PATIENTS

Although a variety of problems may arise, most can be pre-empted by taking a few precautions. For instance, it is worth checking whether a bed is booked at the admission unit. Similarly, if the patient is known to be aggressive, then the police may be approached for assistance.

A patient with a previous history of psychiatric admission or with partial insight, who wishes to avoid compulsory admission, may attempt to do so in a number of ways. The patient may take flight; if this is assessed as being likely to occur, perhaps because of such an incident in the past, the doctor can try to prevent it from happening by carefully explaining the benefits of admission to the patient. Often such a patient may recognize, albeit at an unconscious level, the need for admission. Again, as with certain prisoners in forensic psychiatric assessments, a patient in the community may attempt to give a misleading picture of his or her mental state. However, whereas the former may try to feign mental illness, the latter may endeavour to suppress evidence of mental illness, e.g. by being very guarded in replies to questions, or indeed electively mute. Such a manoeuvre is very likely to fail if the assessment is thorough and includes interviews with relatives and informants, a consideration of the past history, and discussion with others involved in the care of the patient either previously or at the time of the assessment. It should be noted that muteness may in itself be a function of a mental illness, e.g. severe depression or catatonic schizophrenia. In such cases other features of the underlying mental illness will be present and can be elicited.

If a person who is living alone refuses access to his or her home and there is reasonable cause to believe that he or she has been, or is being, ill-treated or neglected, or that he or she is unable to care for himself or herself, e.g. as a result of auditory hallucinations or persecutory delusions, then an application may be made by an Approved Social Worker to a Justice of the Peace for a warrant to be issued to allow the police to enter, by force if need be, and to search for and remove a patient, under

Section 135 of the MHA. Local authorities issue guidance to Approved Social Workers on how to invoke such a power of entry.

There may infrequently be a disagreement between the assessors as to whether compulsory admission is indicated. In such cases it is important that each assessor sets out his or her reasoning clearly during a joint discussion. If there is still no resolution, the professionals present may offer to reassess the patient at a later date. However, it is vital in the event of a decision against compulsory admission that an alternative package of care is implemented to ensure continued support for both the patient and his or her family. The patient should also be encouraged to attend a psychiatric out-patient appointment made for the earliest date possible.

7

PSYCHIATRIC HISTORY-TAKING

PSYCHIATRIC INTERVIEWING

The most important aims of psychiatric interviewing are as follows (Institute of Psychiatry, 1973):

- to *obtain information*;
- to *assess the emotions and attitudes* of the patient;
- the interview (particularly the first interview) plays a *supportive role* and allows an understanding of the patient. This forms the basis of the subsequent working relationship with the patient.

Allow the patient to feel relaxed and uninhibited about talking by fostering a trusting relationship with him or her. Provide a containing environment in which the patient can believe that his or her burdens, including troubling thoughts, can be held by the interviewer.

In general, and particularly at the beginning of the interview, open questions should be used in preference to closed ones; possible responses should not be closed off too soon. It is often helpful to allow the patient to talk without interruption about his or her presenting problem for the first 5 minutes. In due course, when certain details in the history and Mental State Examination need to be established, the interviewer must set the agenda and can home in on these aspects.

When first taking a psychiatric history or carrying out a Mental State Examination, psychiatric trainees may feel uncomfortable about certain aspects, e.g. asking the psychosexual history or enquiring about suicidal thoughts. However, most patients, at least at an unconscious level, expect to be asked about such matters during a psychiatric history-taking. There is no evidence that, by asking questions about suicide, one might place the idea of suicide in the mind of the patient. Rather, the patient may be relieved to be given an opportunity to air these thoughts.

When interviewing a deaf patient who understands sign language, ask for the assistance of a professional signer who has psychiatric experience. If the patient does not speak your language, ask for a professional translator.

POTENTIALLY VIOLENT PATIENTS

If you have to interview a patient who is potentially violent:

- ensure that other members of staff know whom you are interviewing and where;
- ensure that you know the location of panic/alarm buttons and bells;
- sit at right angles to the patient so that he or she has the option of looking away from you;
- sit about a yard away from the patient;
- ensure that you have ready access to the door of the room; ideally the patient should also have such access.

In general, it is helpful if:

- you are aware of your local hospital/ward guidelines on dealing with violence;
- you know how to use panic/alarm buttons and/or personal alarms (check that the battery is not flat);
- you attend a training course in simple breakaway techniques.

Dealing with violence is discussed further in Chapter 24 (Emergencies).

SEXUALLY DISINHIBITED PATIENTS

If you have to interview a patient who may be sexually disinhibited, e.g. a patient with mania, you should ensure that a chaperone, e.g. a psychiatric nurse, of the same sex as the patient is present.

PSYCHIATRIC HISTORY

Ideally this should be derived both from the patient and from other sources of information, including:
- relatives;
- the GP;
- other professionals involved in the case, such as social workers, psychologists, community psychiatric nurses and hostel nursing staff.

The key headings are as follows.

Reason for referral

Complaints

The patient's complaints given in his or her own words. Record also how long each complaint has lasted.

History of presenting illness

A chronological account of the development of each symptom is recorded together with:
- any precipitating factors;
- associated impairments;
- effects on social functioning.

Family history

Record details of parents and siblings, including their:
- current age or age at death;
- occupation;
- health;
- relationship with the patient.

The timing of parental separation and/or divorce, if relevant, should also be recorded.

Family psychiatric history

Record any family history of psychiatric or neurological disorders (e.g. epilepsy), including the nature of the disorder and how and where it has been or is being treated. Record any history of suicide in the family.

Personal history: childhood

Record details of:

- date of birth;
- place of birth;
- abnormalities prior to or at birth;
- whether the birth was premature;
- early developmental milestones;
- childhood health, including any history of 'nervous problems';
- any early emotional stresses, including separation (e.g. because of death) from close relatives such as siblings or parents.

Personal history: education

Record details of:

- age when schooling started;
- types of school attended;
- relationship with peers and teachers;
- any history of truancy or other trouble or difficulties at school;
- qualifications achieved;
- age on leaving school;
- details of higher education, if applicable.

Personal history: occupation(s)

Record:

- summary of occupational history;
- details of promotion/demotion;
- reasons for being sacked repeatedly (e.g. problem drinking), if applicable;
- any other occupational difficulties.

Personal history: psychosexual

Record details (as applicable) of:

- age of menarche;
- any menstrual abnormalities;
- history of pregnancies;
- age of menopause;
- sexual orientation;
- history of sexual abuse;
- history of physical abuse;
- sexual and marital history (including any history of infidelity);
- sexual difficulties.

Personal history: children
Record details (as applicable) of the patient's children, including any disturbances from which they suffer.

Personal history: current social situation
Record the patient's current situation with regard to the following:

- social situation, including the person(s) with whom the patient lives;
- marital status;
- occupation and financial status;
- nature and suitability of accommodation;
- hobbies and social interests.

Past medical history
Record details (as applicable) of the following:

- past and present physical disorders and injuries, including
    their nature,
    where and when they were treated,
    the treatments received;
- medication currently or recently taken;
- side-effects of medication;
- history of hypersensitivity reactions.

Past psychiatric history
Record details (as applicable) of:

- the nature of the illness(es);
- the duration of the illness(es);

- hospital(s) and out-patient department(s) attended;
- treatment(s) received, and any side-effects.

Psychoactive substance use: alcohol

Record details (as applicable) of:

- the number of units of alcohol the patient is currently drinking per week;
- the amount of alcohol consumed in the past;
- any history of withdrawal symptoms;
- any history of physical illnesses, injuries (e.g. road traffic accidents), legal problems (e.g. driving offences) or employment difficulties (e.g. regularly being late for work, resulting in being sacked), which might result from excess alcohol intake.

The CAGE Questionnaire below can be used to screen for alcohol problems (≥ 2 positive answers indicates problem drinking).

C Have you ever felt you should **C**ut down on your drinking?

A Have people **A**nnoyed you by criticizing your drinking?

G Have you ever felt **G**uilty about your drinking?

E Have you ever had a drink first thing in the morning (an **E**ye-opener) to steady your nerves or get rid of a hangover?

Psychoactive substance use: tobacco

Record details (as applicable) of:

- the type of nicotine-containing product used;
- the amount of nicotine-containing product taken;
- any previous history of smoking.

Psychoactive substance use: illicit drugs

Record details (as applicable) of:

- types of drugs taken currently and in the past;
- quantities taken currently and in the past;
- methods of administration used;
- consequences.

Forensic history

Record details (as applicable) of:

- any history of delinquency and criminal activity;
- punishments received (e.g. fines and custodial sentences).

Premorbid personality

The patient's personality consists of their lifelong persistent and enduring characteristics and attitudes, including their way of:

- thinking (cognition);
- feeling (affectivity);
- behaving (impulse control and ways of relating to others and handling interpersonal situations).

If the patient's personality has changed after the onset of a psychiatric disorder, then details of their personality prior to the disorder should be obtained by interviewing both the patient and other informants. Summarize the patient's personality prior to the onset of the psychiatric illness under the following headings:

- attitudes to others in social, family and sexual relationships;
- attitude to self and character;
- moral and religious beliefs and standards;
- predominant mood;
- leisure activities and interests;
- fantasy life – day-dreams and nightmares;
- reaction pattern to stress – including defence mechanisms.

REFERENCES

Institute of Psychiatry 1973: *Notes on eliciting and recording clinical information.* Oxford: Oxford University Press.

8

THE MENTAL STATE EXAMINATION

The Mental State Examination describes the signs of illness exhibited at the time of the interview. Information should also be gathered from other sources, such as the observations of nursing staff in the case of an in-patient, since the patient may not freely admit to all his or her symptomatology.

The main headings of the Mental State Examination follow. Some of these may need to be expanded according to the diagnosis, e.g., in:

- dementia – expand on *mood* and *cognitive state*;
- schizophrenia – expand on *mood*, *abnormal beliefs* and *abnormal experiences*;
- depression – expand on *mood*;
- obsessive-compulsive disorder – expand on *mood* and *thought abnormalities*.

APPEARANCE AND BEHAVIOUR

General appearance

Describe the patient's general appearance and detail any features that may be consistent with a psychiatric disorder, such as:

- self-neglect – a lack of cleanliness in self-care, hair and clothes that have not been looked after (e.g. dementia, psychoactive substance use disorder, schizophrenia, mood disorder);
- evidence of recent weight loss – poorly fitting clothes that appear too loose (e.g. organic disorders such as carcinoma, or depression);
- change in usual appearance – colourful flamboyant clothing (e.g. mania);

- calluses on the dorsum of the hands – may indicate repeated use of the fingers to stimulate the gag reflex in self-induced vomiting (Russell's sign in bulimia nervosa).

The general appearance may indicate the presence of a physical disorder such as Marfan's syndrome, or an endocrinopathy such as hypopituitarism or one of the endocrinopathies mentioned below in the subsection on facial appearance. The appearance may also indicate obesity or cachexia.

Facial appearance

The patient's facial appearance may give clues to the diagnosis. For example:

- organic disorders – e.g. the typical facial appearances of endocrinopathies such as Cushing's disease, hyperthyroidism, hypothyroidism, acromegaly; systemic lupus erythematosus (butterfly rash); mitral valve disease (malar flush);
- depressive disorder – depressive facies with downcast eyes, a vertical furrow in the forehead and downturning of the corners of the mouth;
- mania – the patient may appear euphoric and/or irritable;
- anxiety – may be associated with raised eyebrows, widening of the palpebral fissures, mydriasis and the presence of horizontal furrows in the forehead;
- Parkinsonian side-effects of antipsychotic medication, or actual Parkinson's disease – relatively fixed unchanging facies;
- anorexia nervosa – fine, downy 'lanugo' hair on the sides of the face (as well as other parts of the body which may not be visible until a physical examination is carried out, such as the arms and back);
- bulimia nervosa – the face may appear chubby owing to parotid gland enlargement, and facial oedema may occur because of purgative abuse.

Posture and movements

Particular disorders may be associated with changes in posture and movements:

- Huntington's disease, Gilles de la Tourette's syndrome, and following encephalitis – tics may occur;
- schizophrenia – the following abnormal movements may occur: ambitendency, echopraxia, mannerisms, negativism, posturing, stereotypies, waxy flexibility (cerea flexibilitas);
- depressive disorder – poor eye contact and hunched shoulders;
- mania – increased movements and an inability to sit still may occur;
- anxiety – may be associated with restlessness;
- Parkinsonism – a festinant gait.

Underactivity

Underactivity may occur in:

- stupor – e.g. in epilepsy, catatonic stupor, depressive stupor, manic stupor, hysteria;
- depressive retardation;
- obsessional slowness.

Overactivity

Overactivity may occur in:

- psychomotor agitation;
- hyperkinesis;
- somnambulism (sleep-walking);
- compulsions.

Psychodynamic aspects

Bear in mind the psychodynamic aspects of movements, e.g. the ring sign, in which a married or engaged woman may play with her wedding or engagement ring during the interview because she has anxieties about her relationship.

Social behaviour

Social behaviour may be altered in:

- dementia – e.g. the interviewer may be ignored;

- schizophrenia – e.g. the patient may act bizarrely, aggressively or suspiciously;
- mania – e.g. the patient may be flirtatious and sexually disinhibited.

Rapport

Record the nature of the rapport established with the patient. This may be indicative of the transference and countertransference, as well as the likely compliance of the patient.

SPEECH

Rate

The rate of speech should be recorded. It may be increased in mania.

Disorders in which the rate may be reduced include dementia and depression.

Quantity

Disorders in which the quantity of speech may be increased include mania and anxiety.

Disorders in which the quantity of speech may be decreased include:

- dementia;
- schizophrenia;
- depression.

Articulation

The accent should be taken into account, as it may mistakenly lead to eliciting the following:

- incorrect psychopathology – e.g. the way in which a word is pronounced may cause the interviewer to consider it to be a neologism;
- incorrect diagnosis – e.g. a rapid, pressured and loud manner of speaking (as in some people from New York) may be thought to indicate hypomania, when it may be the normal way of speaking.

Form

The way in which the patient speaks should be recorded. (Content is recorded under *Thought content*.) If there is a disorder in the form of speech, or one is suspected, record a sample of the speech showing this.

MOOD

Mood

Mood is a pervasive and sustained emotion that, in the extreme, markedly colours the person's perception of the world (DSM-III-R). Give an assessment of the quality of the mood that is:

1. objective – based on the:
   - history;
   - appearance;
   - behaviour;
   - posture;
2. subjective – based on the description of the patient in response to questions such as:
   - 'How do you feel in yourself?';
   - 'How do you feel in your spirits?'.

If the patient appears depressed, the presence of depressive thoughts should be probed further, including asking the patient whether he or she has any suicidal thoughts. If these are present, they should be recorded under *Thought content*.

Anxiety

Anxiety is a feeling of apprehension, tension or uneasiness owing to the anticipation of an external or internal danger. If a patient appears subjectively to be suffering from anxiety, enquire about:

1. the types of anxious thoughts;
2. situations which precipitate anxiety;
3. somatic symptoms from the autonomic nervous system and muscle tension, such as:
   - dry mouth;
   - palpitations;

- atypical chest pain;
- tremor;
- sweating;
- tension headaches.

Affect

Affect is a pattern of observable behaviours that is the expression of a subjectively experienced feeling state (emotion). Affect is variable over time, in response to changing emotional states, whereas mood refers to a pervasive and sustained emotion (DSM-III-R). Record the following aspects of the affect of the patient:

- appropriateness;
- constancy;
- reactivity.

THOUGHT CONTENT

Preoccupations

Record any morbid thoughts, preoccupations and worries of the patient. (The patient can be asked 'What are your main worries and preoccupations?'; 'Do these interfere with your concentration and activities, such as sleep?'.)

Obsessions

Record any obsessions of the patient. (A typical screening question may take the form 'Do you keep having certain thoughts that don't make sense despite your trying to avoid them?'.) Obsessions may be accompanied by compulsions (compulsive rituals).

Phobias

Record any phobias of the patient.

Suicidal thoughts

Record any suicidal thoughts. Bear in mind that suicidal thoughts are not confined to depressive episodes. For example, they are also more common in schizophrenia than in the general population.

Homicidal thoughts

Record any homicidal thoughts. (A typical screening question may take the form 'Have you ever felt the wish to harm others?'.) Bear in mind that homicidal thoughts may accompany suicidal thoughts, e.g. in the case of a depressed mother who decides that life is also not worth living for her children, or again, in the case of a married depressed man who decides to kill his wife as well as himself.

ABNORMAL BELIEFS AND INTERPRETATIONS OF EVENTS

Record details of abnormal beliefs and interpretations of events, including overvalued ideas, delusions and delusional perceptions. Such details should include the following:

• content;
• onset;
• degree of intensity;
• degree of rigidity.

ABNORMAL EXPERIENCES

Record details of abnormal experiences, including sensory distortions, sensory deceptions, and disorders of self-awareness (ego disorders).

COGNITIVE STATE

Check the patient's orientation, attention and concentration, memory, general knowledge and intelligence. If the patient is suspected of having an organic cerebral disorder, then carry out further tests of the cognitive state (see the next section, on *Physical examination*).

Orientation

If disorientation is suspected, assess *orientation* in:

- time – e.g. ask the patient to give the time and date;
- place – e.g. ask the patient to give the current location;
- person – e.g. ask the patient questions about his or her name and identity.

Attention and concentration

These can be checked by asking the patient to carry out the serial sevens test (the patient is asked to subtract 7 from 100 and repeatedly to subtract 7 from the remainder as fast as possible, giving the answer at each stage). Record the time taken to reach a remainder less than 7. The correct answers are as follows:

93, 86, 79, 72, 65, 58, 51, 44, 37, 30, 23, 16, 9 and 2.

If this is too difficult, perhaps because the patient has poor arithmetical skills, ask him or her to carry out the serial threes test. If this is too difficult, ask the patient to recite the names of the days of the week or the months of the year backwards:

- Saturday, Friday, Thursday, Wednesday, Tuesday, Monday and Sunday;
- December, November, October, September, August, July, June, May, April, March, February and January.

As concentration is sustained attention, if the patient copes adequately with the serial sevens, there is no need to check attention separately. If there is poor attention, record the presence of distractibility, and also how easily the patient is aroused.

Memory

Assess the following components of memory (and record any mistakes made by the patient):

- immediate recall – e.g. ask the patient to repeat

immediately a sequence of digits (normal range is 5 to 9 digits, mean is 7);
- registration – e.g. ask the patient to repeat immediately a name and address;
- short-term memory – e.g. 5 minutes after the test of registration, ask the patient to repeat the same name and address;
- memory for recent events – e.g. ask the patient to repeat to recall important news items from the previous 2 days;
- long-term memory – e.g. ask the patient to recall his or her date and place of birth.

General knowledge

This can be assessed by asking the patient to name, for example:
- the President of the USA;
- the colours of the national flag;
- five capital cities in a given continent, or five state capitals.

Intelligence

An assessment can be made of whether the patient's intelligence is within the normal range, clinically, from:
- his or her answers to the general knowledge questions;
- his or her responses to questions regarding the history and Mental State Examination thus far; and
- the level of education achieved (from the history).

INSIGHT

If the patient has a psychiatric disorder, the degree of insight into this can be assessed by finding out whether the patient:
- recognizes that he or she is ill;
- accepts that he or she has a psychiatric illness;
- accepts that psychiatric treatment is necessary.

Do not simply record the insight as being absent or present. Instead, explain the degree of insight with reference to the above three criteria. (For example, 'Mr Y had partial insight into his condition in that he recognized he was ill, but did not accept that it was psychiatric in nature and did not accept that he needed treatment'.)

9

PHYSICAL EXAMINATION

DIRECT QUESTIONS

Ask about:
- appetite and weight change (if not already covered in the psychiatric history);
- tiredness and lethargy (if not already covered in the psychiatric history);
- the presence of any lumps;
- fever;
- nocturnal sweating;
- endocrine symptoms, particularly those of hyperthyroidism and hypothyroidism;
- cardiovascular symptoms;
- respiratory symptoms;
- gastrointestinal symptoms;
- genito-urinary symptoms;
- musculoskeletal symptoms;
- neurological symptoms.

INTIMATE EXAMINATIONS AND CHAPERONING

In 1996 the GMC issued guidelines on conducting intimate physical examinations, which can serve as a guide to conducting any physical examinations that involve undressing by the patient:
- explain to the patient that an (intimate) examination needs to be carried out, and why this is so;
- explain what it will involve and obtain permission;
- whenever possible offer a chaperon or invite the patient to bring a relative or friend;

- give privacy to undress and dress;
- keep discussion relevant and avoid personal remarks;
- encourage questions and discussions.

In general, it is highly advisable only to examine a patient physically in the presence of a chaperon.

GENERAL PHYSICAL EXAMINATION

General inspection

In addition to the signs looked for under appearance and behaviour in the Mental State Examination, check specifically for:

- cyanosis – central cyanosis and peripheral cyanosis;
- degree of hydration;
- jaundice – check the sclerae;
- pallor;
- anaemia – check the conjunctivae and skin folds;
- hyperpigmentation – e.g. in Addison's disease;
- ocular signs – e.g. Kayser-Fleischer rings.

Lymph nodes

Check for lymphadenopathy in the following regions:

- neck – palpate from behind the patient;
- axillae (Fig. 9.1e);
- supraclavicular (Fig. 9.1f);
- epitrochlear;
- inguinal;
- abdominal.

Hands

Check the nails for:

- onycholysis – may suggest hyperthyroidism, psoriasis or fungal infection;
- koilonychia – may suggest iron deficiency, syphilis, etc.;

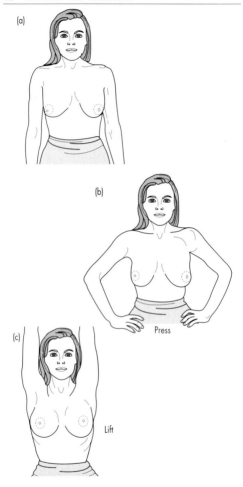

FIGURE 9.1   Breast examination. (a) Inspection of the breasts with the patient sitting up with her arms by her side. (b) Inspection of the breasts with the patient sitting up with her hands pressing down on her hips. (c) Inspection of the breasts with the patient sitting up with her arms elevated.

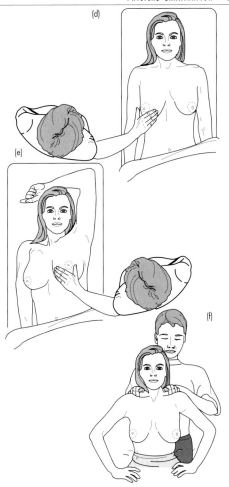

FIGURE 9.1 Breast examination. (d) Palpation of the breasts with the patient lying supine with her arms by her side. (e) Palpation of the breasts and axillae with the patient lying supine with the corresponding arm raised in turn as shown. (f) Palpation of the supraclavicular lymph nodes with the patient sitting up.

- splinter haemorrhages – may be normal or, if the patient is pyrexial, may suggest infective endocarditis;
- clubbing – may occur, for example, in bronchial carcinoma, chronic lung suppuration, hepatic cirrhosis, lymphoma, malabsorption, infective endocarditis, cyanotic congenital cardiac disease, or hyperthyroidism;
- nicotine stains.

Check the palms for:

- palmar crease hyperpigmentation – may occur in Addison's disease;
- palmar crease pallor – may occur in anaemia;
- palmar erythema – may occur in hepatic cirrhosis, polycythaemia or pregnancy;
- Dupuytren's contracture – may occur in hepatic cirrhosis, epilepsy, trauma or ageing.

Breast examination

A breast examination includes (see Fig. 9.1):

- inspection of the breasts with arms raised;
- inspection of the breasts with arms lowered and hands pressing on hips;
- inspection of skin involvement – *peau d'orange*;
- inspection of nipple inversion;
- inspection of nipple discharge;
- palpation.

If a lump is present, note its:

- position;
- size;
- mobility;
- fixity;
- consistency.

Also check for local lymphadenopathy.

Cardiovascular system

Examination of this system includes:

- inspection;
- pulse;
- blood pressure;
- jugular venous pressure;

- palpation of the apex beat and of any parasternal heaving (right ventricular hypertrophy) or thrills;
- auscultation of the heart – heart sounds and any murmurs;
- evidence of peripheral vascular disease or oedema.

Respiratory system
Examination of this system includes:
- inspection, including chest movements;
- palpation of the trachea and chest expansion;
- percussion;
- auscultation;
- vocal resonance.

Gastrointestinal system
Examination of this system includes:
- inspection;
- palpation – including the liver, spleen and kidneys;
- percussion – if there is evidence of ascites;
- auscultation – bowel sounds and bruits.

CRANIAL NERVES

I: Olfactory nerve
Test the ability to differentiate between different smells presented to each nostril.

II: Optic nerve
For each eye, test:
1. visual acuity;
2. visual field;
3. pupils:
   - size;
   - shape;
   - symmetry;
   - response to light (direct and consensual).
Using an ophthalmoscope, check:

- the red reflex;
- evidence of cataracts;
- the retina.

III, IV and VI: Oculomotor, trochlear and abducent nerves
Test these cranial nerves and also disorders of eye movement as a result of, for example, Huntington's disease:

- horizontal movement to the left and right;
- vertical movement upwards and downwards;
- maintainence of gaze in the left, right, upward and downward positions;
- smooth-pursuit eye movements;
- saccadic horizontal and vertical eye movements.

Check for evidence of ptosis, diplopia and nystagmus.

V: Trigeminal nerve
Test:

1. corneal reflex;
2. jaw jerk;
3. sensation in the areas of innervation of:
   - the ophthalmic division;
   - the maxillary division;
   - the mandibular division;
4. motor functioning – ask the patient to open his or her mouth (a lesion leads to deviation to that side).

VII: Facial nerve
Ask the patient to:

- raise his or her eyebrows;
- show his or her teeth;
- identify tastes.

VIII: Vestibulocochlear nerve
Test:

- hearing – ask for a sentence whispered into each ear in turn to be repeated back, while blocking the other ear;

- positional nystagmus.

If hearing is impaired, and this is not caused by a blockage such as ear wax, then carry out:

- Rinne's test – a vibrating tuning fork is held near the external auditory meatus and then pressed on the mastoid, and the patient is asked to say which appears louder;
- Weber's test – apply a vibrating tuning fork to the midline of the head and test for lateralization.

IX: Glossopharyngeal nerve

Test:

- the gag reflex;
- the palatal reflex.

It is only necessary to test sensation in the posterior third of the tongue and in the pharynx if there is reason to suspect a lesion affecting this cranial nerve.

X: Vagus nerve

In order to examine this nerve:

- listen to the patient's speech – vagal or recurrent laryngeal lesions may lead to dysphonia; lesions of the motor component may give the voice a nasal quality;
- inspect the soft palate while the patient is asked to say 'Ah'.

If these examinations are abnormal, inspect the vocal cords.

XI: Accessory nerve

In order to examine this nerve:

- inspect the bulk of the sternomastoid muscles;
- inspect the bulk of the trapezius muscles;
- test the power of each sternomastoid muscle – ask the patient to turn his or her head against resistance;
- test the power of the trapezius muscles – ask the patient to shrug his or her shoulders against resistance.

XII: Hypoglossal nerve
Inspect the tongue for atrophy, fasciculation, and deviation upon protrusion.

MOTOR SYSTEM

Examination of the motor system includes the following aspects.

Inspection
Look in particular for evidence of:
- abnormal posture;
- muscle wasting;
- fasciculation;
- abnormalities of voluntary movements;
- involuntary movements.

Examination of tone
This includes comparing the left and right sides, and checking for clonus.

Examination of muscle power

Co-ordination
Test co-ordination with:
- the finger-nose test;
- the heel-knee test;
- the eyes closed.

In addition, the patient can be asked rapidly and alternately to pronate and supinate the forearm.

Fine movements assessment

Test for apraxias
Tests for apraxias are considered below.

Test for postural arm drift
Ask the patient to close their eyes and maintain their arms outstretched horizontally.

SENSORY SYSTEM

Examination of the sensory system includes the following aspects.

Examination of sensations

Test for the following sensations:

- touch – using cotton wool or paper;
- temperature – hot and cold tubes;
- pain – pin prick;
- deep pain – squeeze muscles and tendons;
- position sense – including a test for Rombergism (ask the patient to stand, feet together, with closed eyes and outstretched arms);
- vibration sense – using a vibrating tuning fork;
- Barber's chair sign – ask the patient to place their chin rapidly on their chest.

Examination of cortical sensory functioning

Test for:

- two-point discrimination – using two pins or a pair of dividers;
- point localization;
- astereognosis – ask the patient to close their eyes, place an object in the patient's hand and ask them to identify;
- agraphaesthesia – ask the patient to close their eyes, trace a letter or number on their palm, and ask them to identify it;
- texture identification – ask the patient to close their eyes, place an object in the patient's hand and ask them to identify the type of material by feel;
- sensory inattention/extinction – ask the patient to close their eyes, and either apply a stimulus (touch or pin prick) to one side of the body or bilaterally and simultaneously apply the same stimulus; ask the patient to identify which side(s) of the body are being touched.

REFLEXES

Tendon reflexes

The following tendon reflexes can be elicited:

- biceps – C5,6;
- triceps – C6,7;

- supinator – C5,6;
- knee – L(2),3,4;
- ankle – S1,2.

Superficial reflexes

The following superficial reflexes can be elicited:

- plantar;
- abdominal;
- cremasteric.

GAIT AND BALANCE

Observe the patient rising from the sitting position and walking. Major disorders of balance, and also lower limb pyramidal weakness, are unlikely to be present if the patient can successfully carry out the stork manoeuvre (ask the patient, with their eyes open, to balance on one leg while folding their arms across their chest).

FRONTAL RELEASE SIGNS

Frontal lobe lesions can lead to:

- grasping – but it may be normal in those aged over 80 years;
- pouting – but it may be normal in those aged over 70 years;
- positive glabellar tap – but it is also positive in many normal elderly people.

FRONTAL EXECUTIVE FUNCTIONS

Verbal fluency

This tests initiation. The patient is asked to recall as many words as possible, as quickly as possible, which begin with the letter F, during a period of 1 minute. The patient is told that proper nouns (e.g. names of people and places) and words derived from or variations of words already given (e.g. plurals and participles) are not counted. This procedure is then repeated for the letters A and S. A total score for all three letters of less than 30 is usually abnormal.

Other tests of verbal fluency may, for example, involve asking the patient to name as many four-legged animals or types of fruit as possible during a period of 1 minute.

Proverbs

This tests abstraction. The patient is asked to interpret a proverb, such as 'A bird in the hand is worth two in the bush' or 'One swallow doesn't make a summer'.

Similarities

This also tests abstraction. The patient is asked to explain the way in which conceptually linked pairs of words are the same, such as:

- orange and pear;
- coat and dress;
- bed and wardrobe;
- poem and statue;
- praise and punishment.

Wisconsin Card Sort Test

This tests response inhibition and set-shifting. Using either a computerized version (perhaps with a touch screen) or a pack of special cards, the patient has to determine the rule for allocating cards and then allocate accordingly. When the rule changes, if the patient has a frontal lesion, then perseverative errors are likely to occur. The rules are based on:

- the number of symbols on the cards;
- the colour of the symbols on the cards;
- the shape of the symbols on the cards.

Alternating sequence

This is not as effective a method of testing response inhibition and set-shifting as the Wisconsin Card Sort Test. An alternating sequence, such as the one shown in Fig. 9.2, is presented to the patient, who is

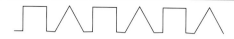

FIGURE 9.2 An alternating sequence which the patient is asked to copy and extend to the right-hand margin of the page.

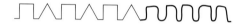

FIGURE 9.3 An attempt by a patient with a frontal lesion to copy and extend the alternating sequence shown in Fig. 9.2. Note the perseveration.

asked to copy it and continue it to the right-hand margin of the page.

If the patient has a frontal lesion, perseveration may occur, as shown in Fig. 9.3.

Luria three-step task

This is another test of response inhibition and set-shifting, which again is not as effective as the Wisconsin Card Sort Test. A sequence of hand positions (fist → edge → palm) is demonstrated to the patient five times, without verbal cues, and the patient is then asked to repeat this sequence. Frontal lesions, particularly those affecting the dominant (usually left) side, impair the ability to carry out this procedure correctly.

Alternating hand movements test

This is another test of response inhibition and set-shifting, which again is not as effective as the Wisconsin Card Sort Test. With outstretched arms, a sequence of hand positions (the fingers of one hand extended + other hand with a clenched fist → alternate positions) is demonstrated to the patient five times, without verbal cues, and the patient is then asked to repeat this sequence. Frontal lesions, particularly those affecting the dominant side, impair the ability to carry out this procedure correctly.

LANGUAGE ABILITY

Spontaneous speech
Examine the patient's spontaneous speech for:
- fluency;
- syntax;
- paraphasias – in which words are almost but not precisely correct;
- neologisms;
- word-finding difficulties;
- dysprosody – in which the normal melody of speech is lost;
- telegraphic speech – in which sentences are abridged with words being missed out;
- jargon aphasia – in which the patient utters incoherent meaningless neologistic speech.

Articulation
The articulation of speech can be tested by asking the patient to repeat a phrase such as 'West Register Street' or 'The Leith police dismisseth us'.

Expressing thoughts
The inability to express thoughts, while understanding remains, occurs in expressive or motor aphasia (also known as Broca's non-fluent aphasia). It can be tested by asking the patient to:
- talk about his or her hobbies;
- write to dictation;
- write a passage spontaneously.

Naming
The ability to name objects, which is impaired in nominal aphasia, can be tested by carrying out a word-finding task such as asking the patient to name objects that are pointed to, such as the nib of a pen or a shoelace, and to name colours pointed to.

Repetition

An inability to repeat in aphasia may occur if perisylvian language areas are affected. A screening task is provided by asking the patient verbally to repeat the following phrase: 'No ifs, ands, or buts'.

Comprehension

Difficulty in comprehending word meanings occurs in receptive or sensory aphasia (also known as Wernicke's fluent aphasia). It can be tested by asking the patient to:

- read a passage;
- explain the passage;
- respond to commands – e.g. 'Touch your right ear with your left hand and then touch my left index finger'; this also screens for right-left disorientation.

Reading

A screening task is provided by asking the patient to carry out the command shown on a piece of paper, such as that in Fig. 9.4.

If there is a specific difficulty in reading, then more specific tests of dyslexia can be carried out.

Writing

A screening task is provided by asking the patient to write a sentence of his or her own choice that makes sense. If there is a specific difficulty in writing, then more specific tests of dysgraphia can be carried out.

HANDEDNESS

If dysfunction in language ability is found, the handedness of the patient should be determined. It is not sufficient simply to ask which hand is used predominantly in writing. For example, some left-handers may have been forced to learn to write with the right hand during childhood. A more accurate picture is obtained by using the Annett Handedness Questionnaire (see Fig. 9.5).

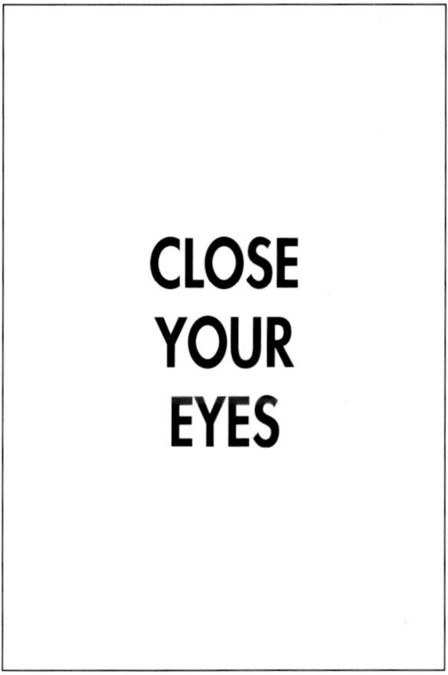

CLOSE
YOUR
EYES

FIGURE 9.4   The patient is asked to carry out the command shown on this piece of paper.

CALCULATION

Acalculia (difficulty with writing, reading and comprehending numbers – often found with aphasia) and anarithmetica (difficulty in carrying out addition, subtraction, multiplication and division in the absence of acalculia – may occur in dementia) can be tested by asking the patient to:

- write out to dictation single digit numbers – e.g. 4, 3, 9, 7;
- write out to dictation numbers with more than one digit – e.g. 54, 46, 682, 1597;
- read aloud written numbers;

Modified version of the Annett Handedness Questionnaire (after Annett 1970)

Which hand do you use:

1. To write a letter legibly?
2. To throw a ball to hit a target?
3. To hold a racket in tennis, squash or badminton?
4. To hold a match while striking it?
5. To cut with scissors?
6. To guide a thread through the eye of a needle (or guide a needle on to thread?)
7. At the top of a broom while sweeping?
8. At the top of a shovel when moving sand?
9. To deal playing cards?
10. To hammer a nail into wood?
11. To hold a toothbrush while cleaning your teeth?
12. To unscrew the lid of a jar?

If you use the right hand for all these actions, are there any one-handed actions for which you use the left hand?

13. With which eye would you look through a telescope?
    (If you are not sure, roll a paper into a tube and look down it.)
14. Which foot would you use to kick a ball?

FIGURE 9.5 A modified version of the Annett Handedness Questionnaire (after Annett, M. 1970: Classification of hand preference by association analysis. *British Journal of Psychology* **61**, 303–21) (reproduced with permission from Puri, B.K., Laking, P.J. and Treasaden, I.H. 1996: *Textbook of psychiatry.* Edinburgh: Churchill Livingstone).

- copy out written numbers;
- point to given written numbers;
- carry out basic mental addition;
- carry out basic mental subtraction;
- carry out basic mental multiplication;
- carry out basic mental division;
- carry out basic written addition;
- carry out basic written subtraction;
- carry out basic written multiplication;
- carry out basic written division;

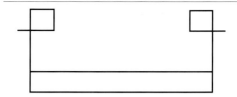

FIGURE 9.6 A typical geometric design that can be used to test non-verbal memory (reproduced with permission from Puri, B.K., Laking, P.J. and Treasaden, I.H. 1996: *Textbook of psychiatry*. Edinburgh: Churchill Livingstone).

- solve an arithmetical problem – e.g. 'If it takes 3 men 4 hours to perform a task, how long would it take 6 men to perform the same task?'.

NON-VERBAL MEMORY

In addition to the tests of verbal memory (dominant hemisphere functions) carried out routinely in the Mental State Examination, tests of non-verbal memory (non-dominant hemisphere functions) can also be performed. A given design, such as that in Fig. 9.6, should be drawn and the patient asked to redraw this:

- immediately – registration and immediate recall;
- after 5 minutes – short-term non-verbal memory.

APRAXIAS

Different types of apraxia (the inability to perform purposive volitional acts, not resulting from paresis, inco-ordination, sensory loss or involuntary movements) can be tested in the following ways.

Constructional apraxia
This is closely associated with visuospatial agnosia, and can be tested by asking the patient to construct

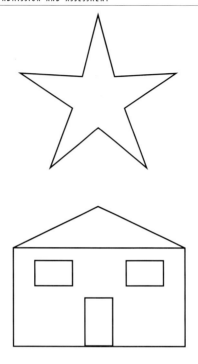

FIGURE 9.7 Two typical figures which the patient can be asked either to construct out of matchsticks or to draw when testing for constructional apraxia and visuospatial agnosia (reproduced with permission from Puri, B.K., Laking, P.J. and Treasaden, I.H. 1996: *Textbook of psychiatry*. Edinburgh: Churchill Livingstone).

a star or some other figure (such as a house) out of matchsticks, or else to draw such a figure (see Fig. 9.7).

The patient can also be asked to copy, at once and from immediate recall, a set of line drawings of progressive difficulty, as shown (from above downwards) in Fig. 9.8.

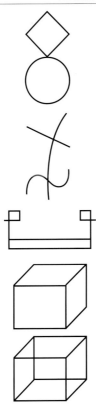

FIGURE 9.8 A set of figures of increasing intricacy which the patient can be asked to copy, both at once and from immediate recall, when testing for constructional apraxia and visuospatial agnosia (reproduced with permission from Puri, B.K., Laking, P.J. and Treasaden, I.H. 1996: *Textbook of psychiatry*. Edinburgh: Churchill Livingstone).

Dressing apraxia
This is tested by asking the patient to put on items of clothing.

Ideomotor apraxia

This is tested by asking the patient to carry out progressively difficult tasks, e.g. touching different parts of the face with specified fingers.

Ideational apraxia

This is tested by asking the patient to carry out a co-ordinated sequence of actions, such as 'Cut this piece of paper in two using the pair of scissors provided and then fold one of the resulting pieces and place it in the envelope'.

Clearly if there is any evidence of risk from the history and Mental State Examination (e.g. the presence of homicidal thoughts), then a potentially dangerous weapon such as a pair of scissors should not be made available.

NEGLECT PHENOMENA, AGNOSIAS AND DISORDERS OF BODY IMAGE

Agnosia is an inability to interpret and recognize the significance of sensory information, which does not result from impairment of the sensory pathways, mental deterioration, disorders of consciousness and attention or, in the case of an object, a lack of familiarity with the object. Neglect phenomena should be tested for in hemiplegia.

Visuospatial agnosia

See constructional apraxia above.

Visual (object) agnosia

A familiar object, which can be seen although not recognized by sight, can be recognized through another modality such as touch or hearing.

Prosopagnosia

This is an inability to recognize faces, sometimes in extreme cases even an inability to recognize the reflection of one's own face. If prosopagnosia is suspected, assess the ability of the patient to:

• describe faces;
• recognize and name faces;

- match faces (portraits or photographs);
- identify people from other features – e.g. their voice.

Agnosia for colours

Here the patient is unable to name colours correctly, although colour sense is still present (e.g. coloured cards can be correctly sorted according to colour).

Simultanagnosia

A picture is presented to the patient who, if simultanagnosia is present, is unable to recognize the overall meaning while nevertheless understanding its individual details.

Agraphognosia or agraphaesthesia

See above.

Anosognosia

If anosognosia is present there is a lack of awareness of disease, particularly of hemiplegia (most often following a right parietal lesion). (A localized distortion of body awareness is sometimes called a coenestopathic state.)

Anosodiaphoria

If this is present there is a correct awareness of hemiplegia, but without a full realization of its severity and implications.

Autotopagnosia

This is the inability to name, recognize or point on command to parts of the body, and it can be tested by asking the patient to:

- move given parts of his or her body on command;
- point to given parts of his or her body on command;
- point to given parts of the examiner's body on command;
- name given parts of his or her body.

Astereognosia
See above.

Finger agnosia
This is the inability to recognize individual fingers, be they one's own or those of another. It can be tested by asking the patient, with his or her eyes closed, to identify which of their fingers has been touched.

Topographical disorientation
This can be tested using a locomotor map-reading task in which the patient is asked to trace out a given route on foot.

Personal neglect
This may manifest itself as neglect of one side of the body. For example, only one side may be combed or shaved. If the frontal eye fields are involved, then ocular and head deviation may occur towards the side of the lesion, and therefore away from the neglected side.

Sensory neglect
Particularly with right-sided lesions, sensory inputs from the contralateral side are ignored:
• visual – visual stimuli from the contralateral side to the cerebral lesion are ignored;
• auditory – auditory stimuli from the contralateral side to the cerebral lesion are ignored;
• tactile – tactile stimuli from the contralateral side to the cerebral lesion are ignored.

Extinction to bilateral simultaneous stimulation
When unilateral stimuli are presented, the patient responds, but he or she fails to do so when stimuli are presented bilaterally and simultaneously.

Extrapersonal (hemispatial) neglect
This is particularly likely to occur following right-sided lesions, and it can be tested by asking the patient to:
• search visually for a given letter or shape amongst a presented array;

- draw in the numbers on a clock-face – the left side of the clock is neglected (following a right-sided lesion), or all 12 numbers are placed on the right side, again neglecting the left side of the clock;
- bisect a straight line – a right-sided lesion may cause the patient to bisect the line to the right of the midpoint, so that the left side is again neglected.

Neglect dyslexia
Right-sided cerebral lesions may result in the left side of individual words or of individual lines being ignored when text is being read out aloud (leading to nonsense).

Neglect dysgraphia
Right-sided cerebral lesions may result in the left side of individual words or of individual lines being ignored when text is being written (leading to nonsense).

Distorted awareness of size and shape
Here a limb, for example, may be felt to be growing larger.

Hemisomatognosis or hemidepersonalization
Here the patient feels that a limb (which is in fact present) is missing.

Phantom limb
This is the continued awareness of the presence of a limb in a patient when that limb has been removed.

Reduplication phenomenon
Here the patient feels that part or all of his or her body has been duplicated.

10

INVESTIGATIONS

Laboratory and diagnostic investigations can serve a number of purposes:
- ruling out an organic cause for the patient's symptomatology;
- routine screening – establishes a baseline and may detect abnormalities not manifested or detected clinically;
- repeat investigations – indicate changes over time and with respect to changes in symptomatology;
- patient evaluation before commencing specific biological therapies such as electroconvulsive therapy and certain types of pharmacotherapy (e.g. prior to starting treatment with lithium);
- follow-up evaluation of treatments (e.g. with lithium);
- research.

FURTHER INFORMATION

In the assessment of a patient it is useful to obtain further information from sources such as:
- relatives;
- the general practitioner;
- other professionals involved with the patient – e.g. social workers, probation officers, teachers;
- previous medical and psychiatric case-notes;
- relevant legal documents.

FIRST-LINE INVESTIGATIONS

First-line investigations that should be routinely carried out for newly admitted in-patients include the following.

Blood tests

These include:

- full blood count;
- urea and electrolytes;
- thyroid function tests;
- liver function tests;
- vitamin B_{12} level, if clinically indicated;
- folate level, if clinically indicated;
- syphilis serology, if clinically indicated.

Urine tests

These include a drug screen.

SECOND-LINE INVESTIGATIONS

Second-line investigations that can be carried out if indicated by the history, Mental State Examination and physical examination may include the following:

- special blood tests – e.g. other endocrine investigations, HIV serology;
- special urine tests – e.g. porphobilinogen, δ-aminolaevulinic acid;
- electroencephalography (EEG);
- psychometric testing;
- structural neuroimaging – e.g. magnetic resonance imaging (MRI), X-ray computerized tomography (CT);
- functional neuroimaging – e.g. magnetic resonance spectroscopy (MRS), positron emission tomography (PET), single-photon emission tomography (SPET), functional magnetic resonance (fMR);
- brain electrical activity mapping (BEAM);
- genetic tests.

TABLE 10.1   Normal ranges for laboratory investigations

Analyte	Reference interval
Blood (venous) biochemistry	
Acid phosphatase (prostatic)	$0-1$ IU L^{-1}
Alanine aminotransferase (ALT)	$5-35$ IU L^{-1}
Albumin	$35-50$ g L^{-1} (non-pregnant)
Alkaline phosphatase	$30-300$ IU L^{-1} (adult)
Amylase	$50-300$ IU L^{-1}
Aspartate transaminase (AST)	$5-35$ IU L^{-1}
Bilirubin (total)	$2-17$ μmol L^{-1}
Calcium (total)	$2.12-2.65$ mmol L^{-1}
Chloride	$95-105$ mmol L^{-1}
Cholesterol (fasting)	$3.6-6.7$ mmol L^{-1}
Copper	$11-24$ μmol L^{-1}
Creatine kinase (CK)	$30-200$ IU L^{-1} (males)
	$30-150$ IU L^{-1} (females)
Folate	$2-20$ μg L^{-1}
γ-glutamyl transpeptidase (γGT, γGTT)	$10-55$ IU L^{-1} (males)
	$5-35$ IU L^{-1} (females)
Glucose (fasting)	$3.5-5.8$ mmol L^{-1}
Growth hormone	$0-20$ mU L^{-1}
Iron	$14-32$ μmol L^{-1} (males)
	$10-30$ μmol L^{-1} (females)
Iron-binding capacity (total)	$54-75$ μmol L^{-1}
Lactate dehydrogenase (LDH)	$100-300$ IU L^{-1}
Magnesium	$0.75-1.05$ mmol L^{-1}
Phosphate (inorganic)	$0.8-1.4$ mmol L^{-1}
Potassium	$3.3-5.0$ mmol L^{-1}
Prolactin	$0-450$ U L^{-1} (males)
	$0-600$ U L^{-1} (females)
Protein (total)	$60-82$ g L^{-1}
Sodium	$133-145$ mmol L^{-1}
Thyroid-binding globulin (TBG)	$7-17$ mg L^{-1}
Thyroid-stimulating hormone (TSH)	$0.5-5.7$ mU L^{-1} (<50 years old)
	0.5 to $(5.7 + x)$ mU L^{-1} ($\geqslant 50$ years old, where x is the number of decades over the age of 40 years)
Thyroxine (T_4)	$70-140$ nmol L^{-1}
Thyroxine (free)	$9-22$ pmol L^{-1}
Triglyceride (fasting)	$0.6-1.7$ mmol L^{-1}
Tri-iodothyronine (T_3)	$1.2-3.0$ nmol L^{-1}

Analyte	Reference interval
Urate	0.12–0.48 mmol L^{-1} (males)
	0.12–0.39 mmol L^{-1} (females)
Urea	2.5–6.7 mmol L^{-1}
Vitamin B$_{12}$ (as serum cyanocobalamin)	160–925 ng L^{-1}

Urine biochemistry
Cortisol (free)	0–280 nmol 24 h^{-1}
Hydroxyindoleacetic acid (HIAA)	16–73 μmol 24 h^{-1}
3-methoxy-4-hydroxymandelic acid (vanillyl mandelic acid, VMA)	16–48 μmol 24 h^{-1}
Potassium	14–120 mmol 24 h^{-1}
Protein	0–150 mg 24 h^{-1}
Sodium	100–250 mmol 24 h^{-1}

Blood (venous) haematology
Erythrocyte sedimentation rate (ESR) (Westergren method)	0–[(age in years)/2] mm h^{-1} (males)
	0–([(age in years) + 10]/2) mm h^{-1} (females)
Haemoglobin	13–18 g dL^{-1} (men)
	11.5–16.5 g dL^{-1} (women)
Mean corpuscular haemoglobin (MCH)	27–32 pg
Mean corpuscular haemoglobin concentration (MCHC)	30–36 g dL^{-1}
Mean corpuscular volume (MCV)	76–98 fL
Packed cell volume (PCV) or haematocrit	0.40–0.54 (men)
	0.35–0.47 (women)
Platelets	150–400 × 10^9 L^{-1}
Prothrombin time	11–15 s
Red cell count	4.5–6.5 × 10^{12} L^{-1} (men)
	3.8–5.8 × 10^{12} L^{-1} (women)
Reticulocytes	10–100 × 10^9 L^{-1} (adults)
White cell count (WCC)	4.0–11.0 × 10^9 L^{-1} (adults)
Neutrophil granulocytes	2.5–7.5 × 10^9 L^{-1} (40–75% WCC)
Lymphocytes	1.0–3.5 × 10^9 L^{-1} (20–45% WCC)
Eosinophil granulocytes	0.04–0.44 × 10^9 L^{-1} (1–6% WCC)
Basophil granulocytes	0–0.10 × 10^9 L^{-1} (0–1% WCC)
Monocytes	0.2–0.8 × 10^9 L^{-1} (2–10% WCC)

II

USE OF RATING SCALES

—

Mini-Mental State Examination

The Mini-Mental State Examination is a commonly used standardized mental test schedule. Despite its limitations, it is useful as a screening tool because of its relatively high inter-rater reliability.

It samples a number of different areas of cognition, including memory, attention, visuospatial ability, etc. If the failure is restricted to one area rather than spread over all areas it has different significance.

The Mini-Mental State Examination was designed to quantify cognitive impairment in older people with dementia, and is reasonably reliable at this task. It is less satisfactory for measuring frontal problems and right hemisphere lesions.

A cut-off point of 24 is a fairly good indicator that someone is suffering from senile dementia, but individuals with above average premorbid intelligence may have Alzheimer's disease and score above 24.

Variables include the following:
- age;
- socio-economic status;
- ethnicity;
- language;
- education – people who are poorly educated will score much lower than individuals who are well educated.

Orientation
- Ask the patient to give the current year, month, day, date and season (score out of 5).

- Ask for the country, county (district), town, hospital and ward (room) (score out of 5).

Registration

- After the examiner has named three common objects (e.g. 'orange, key, ball'), ask the patient to repeat these three words (score out of 3).

Attention and calculation

- Ask the patient to subtract 7 from 100 and 7 from that answer, and so on, as quickly as possible, giving the answer at each stage (the correct answers are 93, 86, 79, 72, 65 – stop the patient after five answers and do not correct him or her if errors are made; score out of 5).
- *Alternatively,* ask the patient to spell the word 'WORLD' backwards (the correct answer is DLROW; score out of 5).

Recall

- Ask the patient to name the three objects learned earlier (score out of 3).

Language

- Ask the patient to name two objects (a pencil and a watch) that are shown to him or her (score out of 2).
- Ask the patient to repeat the sentence 'No ifs, ands or buts' (score out of 1).

Three-stage command

- Present a piece of paper to the patient and say 'Take this paper in your left (or right) hand, fold it in half, and place it on the floor' (score out of 3).

Reading

- Ask the patient to read and obey a written command on a piece of paper that states 'CLOSE YOUR EYES' as shown in Fig. 9.4 (score out of 1).

Writing

- Ask the patient to write a sentence (give it a score of 1 if it is sensible and has a subject and a verb).

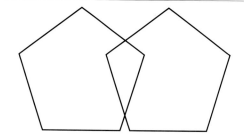

FIGURE 11.1 Overlapping pentagons from the Mini-Mental State Examination.

Construction
• Ask the patient to copy the drawing of intersecting pentagons shown in Fig. 11.1 (score out of 1).

Total score
• The total score of the patient, out of a maximum of 30, is recorded.

Geriatric Depression Scale

Depression in old age is common, underdiagnosed and undertreated, making it an ideal subject for screening. It should be included in the over 75 years screening programme carried out by general practitioners.

There are several screening questionnaires for depression in the elderly which have been shown to be reliable and valid. These include the Self-Care D and the Geriatric Depression Scale (GDS).

The GDS is a 30-question (yes/no) questionnaire which is easy to administer and is acceptable to patients. It can also be shortened to a 15-item scale for speed of administration, and there is a 4-item variant which sacrifices reliability for the sake of speed.

Other important rating scales

General morbidity

- General Health Questionnaire (GHQ) – 60 items, self-administered.
- Hopkins Symptom Checklist (HSC) – 58 items, self-administered.
- Symptom Sign Inventory (SSI) – 80 items, by interviewer.

Diagnostic

- Schedule for Affective Disorders and Schizophrenia (SADS) – 7-point rating scales, semi-structured interview, oriented to Research Diagnostic Criteria (RDC) diagnoses.
- Structured Clinical Interview for DSM-III-R (SCID) – 3-point rating scales, semi-structured interview, oriented to DSM-III-R diagnoses.
- Present State Examination (PSE) – structured interview, associated CATEGO program.
- Brief Psychiatric Rating Scale (BPRS) – semi-structured interview.

Alcohol use

- CAGE Questionnaire – 4 items (**C**ut down, **A**nnoyed, **G**uilty, **E**ye-opener).
- Alcohol Use Inventory (AUI) – 228 items, self-report.

Schizophrenia

- Scale for the Assessment of Positive Symptoms (SAPS) – 5-point rating scales of hallucinations, delusions, bizarre behaviour and positive formal thought disorder.
- Scale for the Assessment of Negative Symptoms (SANS) – 5-point rating scales of affective flattening/blunting, alogia, avolition–apathy, anhedonia–asociality and attention.

Mania

- Manic-State Rating Scale (MRSR) – 26 items, observer rating.

- Bech-Rafaelsen Rating Scale for Mania – 11 items, clinical interview.
- Rating Scale for Mania – 11 items.

Depression
- Hamilton Rating Scale for Depression (HAM-D) – 17 to 24 items, clinical interview.
- Beck Depression Inventory (BDI) – 20 items, self-report.
- Montgomery-Åsberg Depression Rating Scale (MADRS) – 17 items, observer rating.

Anxiety
- Hamilton Rating Scale for Anxiety – 96 items, clinical interview.
- State-Trait Anxiety Inventory (STAI) – 2 × 20 items, self-report.

Suicidal behaviour
- Suicide Intent Scale (SIS) – 15 items, self-report.
- Reasons for Living Inventory (RFL) – 6 factors, self-report.

Personality disorder
- Personality Assessment Schedule (PAS) – yields five diagnostic categories (sociopathic, schizoid, passive-dependent, anankastic and normal).
- Structured Interview for DSM-III-R Personality Disorders (SIDP-R) – yields DSM-III-R Axis II diagnoses.

12

DESCRIPTIVE PSYCHOPATHOLOGY

DISORDERS OF GENERAL BEHAVIOUR

UNDERACTIVITY

Stupor
The key features of stupor, when the term is used in its psychiatric sense, include:
- mutism;
- immobility;
- occasional periods of excitement and over-activity.

Stupor is seen in:
- catatonic stupor;
- depressive stupor;
- manic stupor;
- epilepsy;
- hysteria.

In neurology, the term stupor refers to a patient who responds to pain and loud sounds, and who may exhibit brief monosyllabic utterances, and some spontaneous motor activity takes place.

Depressive retardation
This is a lesser form of psychomotor retardation occurring in depression which, in its extreme form, merges with depressive stupor.

Obsessional slowness
This may occur secondary to repeated doubts and compulsive rituals.

OVERACTIVITY

Psychomotor agitation

A patient with psychomotor agitation manifests:

- excess overactivity – usually unproductive;
- restlessness.

Hyperkinesis

In hyperkinesis, which may be seen in children and adolescents, the following features occur:

- overactivity;
- distractibility;
- impulsivity;
- excitability.

Somnambulism (sleep walking)

A complex sequence of behaviours is carried out by a person who rises from sleep and is not fully aware of his or her surroundings.

Compulsion (compulsive ritual)

This is a repetitive, stereotyped, seemingly purposeful behaviour. It is the motor component of an obsessional thought. Examples of compulsions include:

- checking rituals;
- cleaning rituals;
- counting rituals;
- dressing rituals;
- nymphomania – a compulsive need in the female to engage in sexual intercourse;
- polydipsia – a compulsion to drink water;
- satyriasis – a compulsive need in the male to engage in sexual intercourse;
- trichotillomania – a compulsion to pull out one's hair.

ABNORMAL POSTURE AND MOVEMENTS

Particularly in schizophrenia, but sometimes also in other disorders such as some learning disabilities, the following abnormal movements may occur:

ambitendency, echopraxia, mannerisms, negativism, posturing, stereotypies and waxy flexibility.

Ambitendency

The patient makes a series of tentative incomplete movements when expected to carry out a voluntary action.

Echopraxia

This refers to the automatic imitation by the patient of another person's movements. It occurs even when the patient is asked not to do it.

Mannerisms

These are repeated involuntary movements that appear to be goal directed.

Negativism

This is a motiveless resistance to commands and to attempts to be moved.

Posturing

The patient adopts an inappropriate or bizarre bodily posture continuously for a long time.

Stereotypies

These are repeated regular fixed patterns of movement (or speech) which are not goal directed.

Waxy flexibility (cerea flexibilitas)

There is a feeling of plastic resistance resembling the bending of a soft wax rod as the examiner moves part of the patient's body. That body part then remains 'moulded' by the examiner in the new position.

Tics

These are repeated irregular movements involving a muscle group and may be seen, for example, following encephalitis, in Huntington's disease and in Gilles de la Tourette's syndrome.

Parkinsonism

The features of Parkinsonism include:

- a resting tremor;
- cogwheel rigidity;

- postural abnormalities;
- a festinant gait.

DISORDERS OF SPEECH

DISORDERS OF RATE, QUANTITY AND ARTICULATION

Dysarthria
This is difficulty in the articulation of speech.

Dysprosody
This is speech with the loss of its normal melody.

Logorrhoea (volubility)
This is speech that is fluent and rambling, with the use of many words.

Mutism
This is the complete loss of speech.

Poverty of speech
There is a restricted amount of speech. If the patient replies to questions, he or she may do so with monosyllabic answers.

Pressure of speech
In pressure of speech there is an increase in both the quantity and rate of speech, which is difficult to interrupt.

Stammering
The flow of speech is broken by pauses and the repetition of parts of words.

DISORDERS OF THE FORM OF SPEECH

Circumstantiality
Thinking appears slow, with the incorporation of unnecessary trivial details. However, the goal of thought is eventually reached.

Echolalia
This is the automatic imitation by the patient of another person's speech. It occurs even when the

patient does not understand the speech (which may, for example, be in another language).

Flight of ideas

The speech consists of a stream of accelerated thoughts with abrupt changes from topic to topic, and no central direction. The connections between the thoughts may be based on:

- chance relationships;
- clang associations;
- distracting stimuli;
- verbal associations – e.g. alliteration and assonance.

Neologism

This is either a new word constructed by the patient, or an everyday word used in a special way by the patient.

Passing by the point (vorbeigehen)

The answers to questions, although clearly incorrect, demonstrate that the questions are understood. For example, when asked 'What colour is grass?', the patient may reply 'Blue'. It is seen in the Ganser syndrome, first described in criminals awaiting trial.

Perseveration

In perseveration (of both speech and movement) mental operations are continued beyond the point at which they are relevant. Particular types of perseveration of speech include the following:

- *palilalia* – the patient repeats a word with increasing frequency;
- *logoclonia* – the patient repeats the last syllable of the last word.

Thought-blocking

There is a sudden interruption in the train of thought, before it is completed, leaving a 'blank'. After a period of silence, the patient cannot recall what he or she had been saying or had been thinking of saying.

Disorders (loosening) of association (formal thought disorder)

These occur particularly in schizophrenia, and may be considered to be a schizophrenic language disorder. Examples include *knight's move thinking*, in which there are odd tangential associations between ideas, leading to disruptions in the smooth continuity of the speech, and *schizophasia*, also called *word salad* or *speech confusion*, in which the speech is an incoherent and incomprehensible mixture of words and phrases. Schneider described the following features of formal thought disorder:

- *derailment* – the thought derails on to a subsidiary thought;
- *drivelling* – there is a disordered intermixture of the constituent parts of one complex thought;
- *fusion* – heterogeneous elements of thought are interwoven with each other;
- *omission* – a thought or part of a thought is senselessly omitted;
- *substitution* – a major thought is replaced by a subsidiary thought.

DISORDERS OF EMOTION

DISORDERS OF AFFECT

Affect is a pattern of observable behaviours which is the expression of a subjectively experienced feeling state (emotion), and is variable over time, in response to changing emotional states (DSM-IV).

Blunted affect
In a patient with a blunted affect the externalized feeling tone is severely reduced.

Flat affect
This consists of a total or almost total absence of signs of expression of affect.

Inappropriate affect
This is an affect which is inappropriate to the thought or speech that it accompanies.

Labile affect
A patient with a labile affect has a labile externalized feeling tone which is not related to environmental stimuli.

DISORDERS OF MOOD

Mood is a pervasive and sustained emotion which, in the extreme, markedly colours the person's perception of the world (DSM-IV).

Dysphoria
This is an unpleasant mood.

Depression
This is a low or depressed mood. It may be accompanied by *anhedonia*, in which the ability to enjoy pleasurable activities is lost. In normal *grief* or mourning, the sadness is appropriate to the loss.

Elation
This is an elevated mood or exaggerated feeling of well-being that is pathological. It is seen in mania.

Euphoria
This is a personal and subjective feeling of unconcern and contentment, usually seen after taking opiates or as a late sequel to head injury.

Irritability
This is a liability to outbursts or a state of reduced control over aggressive impulses towards others. It may be a personality trait or it may accompany anxiety. It also occurs in premenstrual syndrome.

Apathy
This is a loss of emotional tone and the ability to feel pleasure, associated with detachment or indifference.

Alexithymia

This consists of difficulty in the awareness of or description of one's emotions.

DISORDERS RELATED TO ANXIETY

Anxiety

This is a feeling of apprehension, tension or uneasiness due to the anticipation of an external or internal danger. Types of anxiety include:

- *phobic anxiety* – in which the focus of the anxiety is avoided (phobias are a disorder of thought content);
- *free-floating anxiety* – in which the anxiety is pervasive and unfocused;
- *panic attacks* – in which anxiety is experienced in acute, episodic, intense attacks and may be accompanied by physiological symptoms.

Fear

This is anxiety caused by a realistic danger that is recognized at a conscious level.

Agitation

In agitation there is excessive motor activity associated with a feeling of inner tension.

Tension

In tension there is an unpleasant increase in psychomotor activity.

DISORDERS OF THOUGHT CONTENT

PREOCCUPATIONS

Hypochondriasis

This is a preoccupation with a fear of having a serious illness, which is not based on real organic pathology but instead on an unrealistic interpretation of physical signs or sensations as being abnormal.

Monomania
This is a pathological preoccupation with a single object.

Egomania
This is a pathological preoccupation with oneself.

OBSESSIONS

Obsessions are repetitive senseless thoughts which are recognized as irrational by the patient, and which are unsuccessfully resisted. Themes include:

- aggression;
- dirt and contamination;
- fear of causing harm;
- religious themes;
- sexual themes.

PHOBIAS

A phobia is a persistent irrational fear of an activity, object or situation, which leads to avoidance. The fear is out of proportion to the real danger and cannot be reasoned away, as it is not under voluntary control. Some types of phobia include the following:

1. *acrophobia* – fear of heights;
2. *agoraphobia* – literally 'a fear of the market-place', it is a syndrome with a generalized high level of anxiety about, or avoidance of, places or situations from which escape might be difficult, or embarrassing, or in which help might not be available in the event of having a panic attack or panic-like symptoms. Objects of fear may include:
   - crowds;
   - open and closed spaces;
   - shopping;
   - social situations;
   - travelling by public transport;
3. *algophobia* – fear of pain;
4. *claustrophobia* – fear of closed spaces;

5. *social phobia* – fear of personal interactions in a public setting, such as:
   - public speaking;
   - eating in public;
   - meeting people;
6. *specific (simple) phobia* – fear of discrete objects (e.g. snakes) or situations;
7. *xenophobia* – fear of strangers;
8. *zoophobia* – fear of animals.

Phobias of internal stimuli

These include obsessive phobias and illness phobias, which overlap with hypochondriasis.

ABNORMAL BELIEFS AND INTERPRETATIONS OF EVENTS

OVERVALUED IDEAS

An overvalued idea is an unreasonable and sustained intense preoccupation maintained with less than delusional intensity – that is, the patient is able to acknowledge the possibility that the belief may not be true. The idea or belief held is demonstrably false and is not one that is normally held by others of the person's subculture. There is a marked associated emotional investment.

DELUSIONS

A delusion is a false belief based on incorrect inference about external reality that is firmly sustained despite what almost everyone else believes, and despite what constitutes incontrovertible and obvious proof or evidence to the contrary. The belief is not one that is ordinarily accepted by other members of the person's culture or subculture (e.g. it is not an article of religious faith). When a false belief involves a value judgement, it is regarded as a delusion only when the judgement is so extreme as to defy credibility (DSM-IV).

Mood-congruent delusion

In a mood-congruent delusion the content of the delusion is appropriate to the mood of the patient.

Mood-incongruent delusion

In a mood-incongruent delusion the content of the delusion is not appropriate to the mood of the patient.

Primary delusion

This is a delusion that arises fully formed without any discernible connection with previous events. It may be preceded by a *delusional mood* in which the patient is aware of something strange and threatening happening.

Bizarre delusion

This is a delusion involving a phenomenon that the person's culture would regard as totally implausible.

Delusional jealousy (pathological jealousy; Othello syndrome; delusion of infidelity)

This is a delusion that one's sexual partner is unfaithful.

Delusion of being controlled

This is a delusion in which feelings, impulses, thoughts or actions of the patient are experienced as being under the control of some external force, rather than under his or her own control.

Delusion of doubles (l'illusion de sosies)

This is a delusion that a person known to the patient has been replaced by a double. It is seen in Capgras' syndrome.

Delusion of poverty

This is a delusion that one is in poverty.

Delusion of reference

This is a delusion in which events, objects or other people in the patient's immediate environment have a particular and unusual significance. These delusions are usually of a negative or pejorative nature, but may also be grandiose in content (DSM-IV). When similar thoughts are held with less than delusional intensity they are *ideas of reference*.

Delusion of self-accusation
This is a delusion of one's guilt.

Erotomania (de Clérambault's syndrome)
This is a delusion that another person, usually of higher status, is deeply in love with the patient.

Grandiose delusion
This is a delusion of inflated worth, power, knowledge, identity, or special relationship to a deity or famous person.

Passivity phenomenon
This is a delusional belief that an external agency is controlling aspects of the self which are normally entirely under one's own control. Passivity phenomena include:

1. *thought alienation* – the patient believes that his or her thoughts are under the control of an outside agency or that others are participating in his or her thinking. It includes:
   - *thought insertion* – the delusion that certain of one's thoughts are not one's own, but rather are inserted into one's mind by an external agency;
   - *thought withdrawal* – the delusion that one's thoughts are being removed from one's mind by an external agency;
   - *thought broadcasting* – the delusion that one's thoughts are being broadcast out loud so that they can be perceived by others;
2. *made feelings* – the delusional belief that one's own free will has been removed and that an external agency is controlling one's feelings;
3. *made impulses* – the delusional belief that one's own free will has been removed and that an external agency is controlling one's impulses;

4. *made actions* – the delusional belief that one's own free will has been removed and that an external agency is controlling one's actions;
5. *somatic passivity* – the delusional belief that one is a passive recipient of somatic or bodily sensations from an external agency.

Persecutory (querulant) delusion
A delusion in which the central theme is that one (or someone to whom one is close) is being attacked, harassed, cheated, persecuted or conspired against (DSM-IV).

Somatic delusion
A delusion whose main content pertains to the appearance or functioning of one's body (DSM-IV).

DELUSIONAL PERCEPTION

In a delusional perception the patient attaches a new and delusional significance to a familiar real perception without any logical reason.

ABNORMAL EXPERIENCES

SENSORY DISTORTIONS

Hyperaesthesias
These are changes in sensory perception in which there is an increased intensity of sensation. *Hyperacusis* is an increased sensitivity to sounds.

Hypoaesthesias
These are changes in sensory perception in which there is a decreased intensity of sensation. *Hypoacusis* is a decreased sensitivity to sounds.

Changes in quality
Changes in quality of sensations occur particularly with visual stimuli, giving rise to *visual distortions.* Colourings of visual perceptions include:

• *chloropsia* – green;

- *erythropsia* – red;
- *xanthopsia* – yellow.

Dysmegalopsia

Changes in spatial form include:

- *macropsia* – objects are perceived as larger or nearer than is actually the case;
- *micropsia* – objects are perceived as smaller or further away than is actually the case.

SENSORY DECEPTIONS

Illusions

An illusion is a false perception of a real external stimulus.

Hallucinations

An hallucination is a false sensory perception in the absence of a real external stimulus. A hallucination is perceived as being located in objective space and as having the same realistic qualities as normal perceptions. It is not subject to conscious manipulation, and only indicates a psychotic disturbance when there is also impaired reality testing. Hallucinations can be mood congruent or mood incongruent. Types of hallucination include:

1. *auditory*;
2. *autoscopy (phantom mirror image)* – the patient sees himself or herself and knows that it is him or her;
3. *extracampine* – the hallucination occurs outside the patient's sensory field (e.g. a patient was aware of the presence of Adolf Hitler, but always just out of his field of view);
4. *functional* – the stimulus causing the hallucination is experienced in addition to the hallucination itself (e.g. a patient only heard an hallucinatory voice whenever the toilet was flushed);
5. *gustatory*;
6. *hallucinosis* – hallucinations (usually auditory) occur in clear consciousness;

7. *hypnagogic* – the hallucination (usually visual or auditory) occurs while the patient is falling asleep;

8. *hypnopompic* – the hallucination (usually visual or auditory) occurs while the patient is waking from sleep;

9. *olfactory*;

10. *reflex* – a stimulus in one sensory field leads to a hallucination in another sensory field;

11. *somatic* – somatic hallucinations include:
    - *tactile (haptic)* hallucinations – superficial and usually involving sensations on or just beneath the skin in the absence of a real stimulus; these include the sensation of insects crawling under the skin (*formication*);
    - *visceral* hallucinations of deep sensations;

12. *trailing phenomenon* – moving objects are seen as a series of discrete discontinuous images;

13. *visual.*

Pseudohallucinations

A pseudohallucination is a form of imagery that arises in the subjective inner space of the mind. It lacks the substantiality of normal perceptions, and occupies subjective space rather than objective space. It is not subject to conscious manipulation. An *eidetic image* is a vivid and detailed reproduction of a previous perception (a 'photographic memory'). In *pareidolia*, vivid imagery occurs without conscious effort while looking at a poorly structured background (e.g. seeing the image of a person superimposed on a fire).

DISORDERS OF SELF-AWARENESS (EGO DISORDERS)

These include disturbances of:

1. awareness of self-activity, including:
   - *depersonalization* – one feels that one is altered or not real in some way;

- *derealization* – one's surroundings do not seem real;
2. the immediate awareness of self-unity;
3. the continuity of self;
4. the boundaries of the self.

COGNITIVE DISORDERS

DISORIENTATION

This is a disturbance of orientation in time, place or person.

DISORDERS OF ATTENTION

Distractibility
A distractible subject's attention is drawn too frequently to unimportant or irrelevant external stimuli.

Selective inattention
In selective inattention, anxiety-provoking stimuli are blocked out.

DISORDERS OF MEMORY

Amnesia
This is the inability to recall past experiences.

Hypermnesia
In hypermnesia the degree of retention and recall is exaggerated.

Paramnesia
A paramnesia is a distorted recall leading to falsification of memory. Paramnesias include:
- *confabulation* – gaps in memory are unconsciously filled with false memories;
- *déjà vu* – the subject feels that the current situation has been seen or experienced before;
- *déjà entendu* – the illusion of auditory recognition;
- *déjà pensé* – the illusion of recognition of a new thought;

- *jamais vu* – the illusion of failure to recognize a familiar situation;
- *retrospective falsification* – false details are added to the recollection of an otherwise real memory.

DISORDERS OF INTELLIGENCE

Learning disability (mental retardation)
Learning difficulty or mental retardation is classified by DSM-IV and ICD-10 according to the intelligence quotient (IQ) of the subject:

- $50 \leq IQ \leq 70$ ($50 \leq IQ \leq 69$ in ICD-10) – *mild* mental retardation;
- $35 \leq IQ \leq 49$ – *moderate* mental retardation;
- $20 \leq IQ \leq 34$ – *severe* mental retardation;
- $IQ < 20$ – *profound* mental retardation.

Dementia
This is a global organic impairment of intellectual functioning without impairment of consciousness.

Pseudodementia
Pseudodementia resembles dementia clinically, but is not organic in origin.

DISORDERS OF CONSCIOUSNESS

Levels of consciousness
The *neurological* terms used to describe progressively more unconscious levels are:

- *somnolence (drowsiness)* – a subject who is drowsy or somnolent can be awoken by mild stimuli and will be able to speak comprehensibly, albeit perhaps for only a little while, before falling asleep again;
- *stupor* – a stuporose patient responds to pain and loud sounds; brief monosyllabic utterances and some spontaneous motor activity may occur;
- *semi-coma* – a semi-comatose patient will withdraw from the source of pain, but spontaneous motor activity does not take place;

- *deep coma* – no response can be elicited and there is no response to deep pain, nor is there any spontaneous movement; tendon, pupillary and corneal reflexes are usually absent;
- *death*.

Clouding of consciousness
The patient is drowsy and does not react completely to stimuli. There is disturbance of attention, concentration, memory, orientation and thinking.

Delirium
The patient is bewildered, disoriented and restless. There may be associated fear and hallucinations. Variations include:

- *oneiroid state* – a dream-like state in a patient who is not asleep;
- *torpor* – the patient is drowsy and readily falls asleep;
- *twilight state* – a prolonged oneiroid state of disturbed consciousness with hallucinations.

Fugue
This is a state of wandering from the usual surroundings, in which there is also loss of memory.

APHASIAS

Receptive (sensory) aphasia (Wernicke's fluent aphasia)
Difficulty is experienced in comprehending the meaning of words. Types include:

- *agnosic alexia* – words can be seen but cannot be read;
- *pure word deafness* – words that are heard cannot be comprehended;
- *visual asymbolia* – words can be transcribed but cannot be read.

Intermediate aphasia
Types of intermediate aphasia include:

- *central (syntactical) aphasia* – there is difficulty in arranging words in their proper sequence;

- *nominal aphasia* – there is difficulty in naming objects.

Expressive (motor) aphasia (Broca's non-fluent aphasia)
This refers to difficulty in expressing thoughts in words, while comprehension remains.

Global aphasia
Both receptive aphasia and expressive aphasia are present at the same time.

Jargon aphasia
The patient utters incoherent meaningless neologistic speech.

APRAXIAS AND AGNOSIAS

APRAXIAS

Apraxia is an inability to perform purposive volitional acts, which does not result from paresis, incoordination, sensory loss or involuntary movements. It may be considered to be the motor equivalent of agnosia. Types of apraxia include:

- *constructional apraxia* – difficulty in constructing objects or copying drawings; it is closely associated with *visuospatial agnosia*, and some authorities treat the two as being essentially the same;
- *dressing apraxia* – difficulty in putting on one's clothes correctly;
- *ideomotor apraxia* – difficulty in carrying out progressively more difficult tasks, e.g. touching different parts of the face with specified fingers;
- *ideational apraxia* – difficulty in carrying out a coordinated sequence of actions.

AGNOSIAS AND DISORDERS OF BODY IMAGE

Agnosia is an inability to interpret and recognize the significance of sensory information, which does not result from impairment of the sensory pathways, mental deterioration, disorders of consciousness and attention or, in the case of an object, a lack of familiarity with that object. Types of agnosia and disorders of body image include:

- *visuospatial agnosia* – see *constructional apraxia* above;
- *visual (object) agnosia* – a familiar object, which can be seen although not recognized by sight, can be recognized through another modality such as touch or hearing;
- *prosopagnosia* – an inability to recognize faces; in the *mirror sign*, which may occur in advanced Alzheimer's disease, a patient may misidentify his or her own mirrored reflection;
- *agnosia for colours* – the patient is unable to name colours correctly, although colour sense is still present;
- *simultanagnosia* – the patient is unable to recognize the overall meaning of a picture, although its individual details are understood;
- *agraphognosia or agraphaesthesia* – the patient is unable to identify, with closed eyes, numbers or letters traced on his or her palm;
- *anosognosia* – there is a lack of awareness of disease, particularly of hemiplegia (most often following a right parietal lesion);
- *coenestopathic state* – a localized distortion of body awareness;
- *autotopagnosia* – the inability to name, recognize or point on command to different parts of the body;
- *astereognosia* – objects cannot be recognized by palpation;
- *finger agnosia* – the patient is unable to recognize individual fingers, be they his or her own or those of another person;
- *topographical disorientation* – this can be tested by using a locomotor map-reading task in which the patient is asked to trace out a given route by foot;
- *distorted awareness of size and shape* – e.g. a limb may be felt to be growing larger;

- *hemisomatognosis or hemidepersonalization* – the patient feels that a limb (which is in fact present) is missing;
- *phantom limb* – the continued awareness of the presence of a limb that has been removed;
- *reduplication phenomenon* – the patient feels that part or all of his or her body has been duplicated.

13

CLASSIFICATION SYSTEMS — ICD-10 AND DSM-IV

ICD-10

Organic, including symptomatic, mental disorders

F00 Dementia in Alzheimer's disease

F01 Vascular dementia

F02 Dementia in other diseases classified elsewhere

F03 Unspecified dementia

F04 Organic amnesic syndrome, not induced by alcohol and other psychoactive substances

F05 Delirium, not induced by alcohol and other psychoactive substances

F06 Other mental disorders due to brain damage and dysfunction and to physical disease

F07 Personality and behavioural disorders due to brain disease, damage and dysfunction

F09 Unspecified organic or symptomatic mental disorder

Mental and behavioural disorders due to psychoactive substance use

F10 Mental and behavioural disorders due to use of alcohol

F11 Mental and behavioural disorders due to use of opioids

F12 Mental and behavioural disorders due to use of cannabinoids

F13 Mental and behavioural disorders due to use of sedatives or hypnotics

F14 Mental and behavioural disorders due to use of cocaine

F15 Mental and behavioural disorders due to use of other stimulants, including caffeine

F16 Mental and behavioural disorders due to use of hallucinogens

F17 Mental and behavioural disorders due to use of tobacco

F18 Mental and behavioural disorders due to use of volatile solvents

F19 Mental and behavioural disorders due to multiple drug use and use of other psychoactive substances

Schizophrenia, schizotypal and delusional disorders
F20 Schizophrenia
F21 Schizotypal disorder
F22 Persistent delusional disorders
F23 Acute and transient psychotic disorders
F24 Induced delusional disorder
F25 Schizoaffective disorders
F28 Other non-organic psychotic disorders
F29 Unspecified non-organic psychosis

Mood (affective) disorders
F30 Manic episode
F31 Bipolar affective disorder
F32 Depressive episode
F33 Recurrent depressive disorder
F34 Persistent mood (affective) disorders
F35 Other mood (affective) disorders
F39 Unspecified mood (affective) disorder

Neurotic, stress-related and somatoform disorders
F40 Phobic anxiety disorders
F41 Other anxiety disorders
F42 Obsessive-compulsive disorder
F43 Reaction to severe stress, and adjustment disorders
F44 Dissociative (conversion) disorders
F45 Somatoform disorders
F48 Other neurotic disorders

*Behavioural syndromes associated with physiological
disturbances and physical factors*

F50 Eating disorders

F51 Non-organic sleep disorders

F52 Sexual dysfunction, not caused by organic
disorder or disease

F53 Mental and behavioural disorders associated
with the puerperium, not elsewhere classified

F54 Psychological and behavioural factors
associated with disorders or diseases classified
elsewhere

F55 Abuse of non-dependence-producing
substances

F59 Unspecified behavioural syndromes associated
with physiological disturbances and physical
factors

Disorders of adult personality and behaviour

F60 Specific personality disorders

F61 Mixed and other personality disorders

F62 Enduring personality changes, not attributable
to brain damage and disease

F63 Habit and impulse disorders

F64 Gender identity disorders

F65 Disorders of sexual preference

F66 Psychological and behavioural disorders
associated with sexual development and
orientation

F68 Other disorders of adult personality and
behaviour

F69 Unspecified disorder of adult personality and
behaviour

Mental retardation

F70 Mild mental retardation

F71 Moderate mental retardation

F72 Severe mental retardation

F73 Profound mental retardation

F78 Other mental retardation

F79 Unspecified mental retardation

Disorders of psychological development

F80 Specific developmental disorders of speech and language

F81 Specific developmental disorders of scholastic skills

F82 Specific developmental disorder of motor function

F83 Mixed specific developmental disorders

F84 Pervasive developmental disorders

F88 Other disorders of psychological development

F89 Unspecified disorder of psychological development

Behavioural and emotional disorders with onset usually occurring in childhood and adolescence

F90 Hyperkinetic disorders

F91 Conduct disorders

F92 Mixed disorders of conduct and emotions

F93 Emotional disorders with onset specific to childhood

F94 Disorders of social functioning with onset specific to childhood and adolescence

F95 Tic disorders

F98 Other behavioural and emotional disorders with onset usually occurring in childhood and adolescence

Unspecified mental disorder

F99 Mental disorder, not otherwise specified

DSM-IV

The fourth edition of the *Diagnostic and Statistical Manual of Mental Disorders (DSM-IV)*, published by the American Psychiatric Association in 1994, is a multiaxial classification with the following five axes:

Axis I   Clinical disorders
          Other conditions that may be a focus of clinical attention

Axis II   Personality disorders
           Mental retardation

Axis III   General medical conditions

Axis IV   Psychosocial and environmental problems

Axis V   Global assessment of functioning

In the following summary, NOS denotes 'not otherwise specified'. Subtypes are indicated by the use of the letter x in the numerical codes (indicating that a specific code number is required).

Axis I: clinical disorders; other conditions that may be a focus of clinical attention

Disorders usually first diagnosed in infancy, childhood or adolescence

(excluding mental retardation, which is diagnosed on Axis II)

Learning disorders
- 315.00 Reading Disorder
- 315.1 Mathematics Disorder
- 315.2 Disorder of Written Expression
- 315.9 Learning Disorder NOS

Motor skills disorder
- 315.4 Developmental Co-ordination Disorder

Communication disorders
- 315.31 Expressive Language Disorder
- 315.31 Mixed Receptive-Expressive Language Disorder
- 315.39 Phonological Disorder
- 307.0 Stuttering
- 307.9 Communication Disorder NOS

Pervasive developmental disorders
- 299.00 Autistic Disorder
- 299.80 Rett's Disorder
- 299.10 Childhood Disintegrative Disorder
- 299.80 Asperger's Disorder
- 299.80 Pervasive Developmental Disorder NOS

Attention-deficit and disruptive behavior disorders
- 314.xx Attention-Deficit/Hyperactivity Disorder, where xx is

    .01 Combined Type
    .00 Predominantly Inattentive Type
    .01 Predominantly Hyperactive-Impulsive Type
- 314.9 Attention-Deficit/Hyperactivity Disorder
  NOS
- 312.8 Conduct Disorder
      Childhood-Onset Type
      Adolescent-Onset Type
- 313.81 Oppositional Defiant Disorder
- 312.9 Disruptive Behavior Disorder NOS

Feeding and eating disorders of infancy or early childhood
- 307.52 Pica
- 307.53 Rumination Disorder
- 307.59 Feeding Disorder of Infancy or Early
  Childhood

Tic disorders
- 307.23 Tourette's Disorder
- 307.22 Chronic Motor or Vocal Tic Disorder
- 307.21 Transient Tic Disorder
      Single Episode
      Recurrent
- 307.20 Tic Disorder NOS

Elimination disorders
- 787.6 Encopresis With Constipation and
  Overflow Incontinence
- 307.7 Encopresis Without Constipation and
  Overflow Incontinence
- 307.6 Enuresis (Not Due to a General Medical
  Condition)
      Nocturnal Only
      Diurnal Only
      Nocturnal and Diurnal

Other disorders of infancy, childhood or adolescence
- 309.21 Separation Anxiety Disorder
      Specify if Early Onset
- 313.23 Selective Mutism
- 313.89 Reactive Attachment Disorder of Infancy
  or Early Childhood

Inhibited Type
Disinhibited Type
- 307.3 Stereotypic Movement Disorder
  Specify if With Self-Injurious Behavior
- 313.9 Disorder of Infancy, Childhood or
  Adolescence NOS

Delirium, dementia, and amnestic and other cognitive disorders
Delirium
- 293.0 Delirium Due to. . .[Indicate the General
  Medical Condition]
- ---.- Substance Intoxication Delirium (refer to
  Substance-Related Disorders)
- ---.- Substance Withdrawal Delirium (refer to
  Substance-Related Disorders)
- ---.- Delirium Due to Multiple Etiologies
- 780.09 Delirium NOS
Dementia
- 290.xx Dementia of the Alzheimer's Type, With
  Early Onset, where xx is
    .10 Uncomplicated
    .11 With Delirium
    .12 With Delusions
    .13 With Depressed Mood
    Specify if: With Behavioral Disturbance
- 290.xx Dementia of the Alzheimer's Type, With
  Late Onset, where x(x) is
    .0 Uncomplicated
    .3 With Delirium
    .20 With Delusions
    .21 With Depressed Mood
    Specify if: With Behavioral Disturbance
- 290.xx Vascular Dementia, where xx is
    .40 Uncomplicated
    .41 With Delirium
    .42 With Delusions
    .43 With Depressed Mood
    Specify if: With Behavioral Disturbance

- Dementia due to other general medical conditions
    - 294.9 Dementia Due to HIV Disease
    - 294.1 Dementia Due to Head Trauma
    - 294.1 Dementia Due to Parkinson's Disease
    - 294.1 Dementia Due to Huntington's Disease
    - 290.10 Dementia Due to Pick's Disease
    - 290.10 Dementia Due to Creutzfeldt-Jakob Disease
    - 294.1 Dementia Due to. . .[Indicate other General Medical Condition]
    - ---.- Substance-Induced Persisting Dementia
    - ---.- Dementia Due to Multiple Etiologies
    - 294.8 Dementia NOS

Amnestic disorders
- 294.0 Amnestic Disorder Due to. . .[Indicate General Medical Condition]
    - Transient
    - Chronic
- ---.- Substance-Induced Persisting Amnestic Disorder (refer to Substance-Related Disorders)
- 294.8 Amnestic Disorder NOS

Other cognitive disorders
- 294.9 Cognitive Disorder NOS

Mental disorders due to a general medical condition

Substance-related disorders
Alcohol-related disorders
- 303.90 Alcohol Dependence
- 305.00 Alcohol Abuse
- 303.00 Alcohol Intoxication
- 291.8 Alcohol Withdrawal
    - Specify if: With Perceptual Disturbances
- 291.0 Alcohol Intoxication Delirium
- 291.0 Alcohol Withdrawal Delirium
- 291.2 Alcohol-Induced Persisting Dementia
- 291.1 Alcohol-Induced Persisting Amnestic Disorder
- 291.x Alcohol-Induced Psychotic Disorder, where x is

.5 With Delusions
.3 With Hallucinations
- 291.8 Alcohol-Induced Mood Disorder
- 291.8 Alcohol-Induced Anxiety Disorder
- 291.8 Alcohol-Induced Sexual Dysfunction
- 291.8 Alcohol-Induced Sleep Disorder
- 291.9 Alcohol-Related Disorder NOS

Amphetamine (or amphetamine-like)-related disorders

- 304.40 Amphetamine Dependence
- 305.70 Amphetamine Abuse
- 292.89 Amphetamine Intoxication
    Specify if: With Perceptual Disturbances
- 292.0 Amphetamine Withdrawal
- 292.81 Amphetamine Intoxication Delirium
- 292.xx Amphetamine-Induced Psychotic Disorder, where xx is
    .11 With Delusions
    .12 With Hallucinations
- 292.84 Amphetamine-Induced Mood Disorder
- 292.89 Amphetamine-Induced Anxiety Disorder
- 292.89 Amphetamine-Induced Sexual Dysfunction
- 292.89 Amphetamine-Induced Sleep Disorder
- 292.9 Amphetamine-Related Disorder NOS

Caffeine-related disorders

- 305.90 Caffeine Intoxication
- 292.89 Caffeine-Induced Anxiety Disorder
- 292.89 Caffeine-Induced Sleep Disorder
- 292.9 Caffeine-Related Disorder NOS

Cannabis-related disorders

- 304.30 Cannabis Dependence
- 305.20 Cannabis Abuse
- 292.89 Cannabis Intoxication
    Specify if: With Perceptual Disturbances
- 292.81 Cannabis Intoxication Delirium
- 292.xx Cannabis-Induced Psychotic Disorder, where xx is
    .11 With Delusions
    .12 With Hallucinations

- 292.89 Cannabis-Induced Anxiety Disorder
- 292.9 Cannabis-Related Disorder NOS

Cocaine-related disorders
- 304.20 Cocaine Dependence
- 305.60 Cocaine Abuse
- 292.89 Cocaine Intoxication
    Specify if: With Perceptual Disturbances
- 292.0 Cocaine Withdrawal
- 292.81 Cocaine Intoxication Delirium
- 292.xx Cocaine-Induced Psychotic Disorder,
  where xx is
    .11 With Delusions
    .12 With Hallucinations
- 292.84 Cocaine-Induced Mood Disorder
- 292.89 Cocaine-Induced Anxiety Disorder
- 292.89 Cocaine-Induced Sexual Dysfunction
- 292.89 Cocaine-Induced Sleep Disorder
- 292.9 Cocaine-Related Disorder NOS

Hallucinogen-related disorders
- 304.50 Hallucinogen Dependence
- 305.30 Hallucinogen Abuse
- 292.89 Hallucinogen Intoxication
- 292.89 Hallucinogen Persisting Perception
  Disorder (Flashbacks)
- 292.81 Hallucinogen Intoxication Delirium
- 292.xx Hallucinogen-Induced Psychotic
  Disorder, where xx is
    .11 With Delusions
    .12 With Hallucinations
- 292.84 Hallucinogen-Induced Mood Disorder
- 292.89 Hallucinogen-Induced Anxiety Disorder
- 292.9 Hallucinogen-Related Disorder NOS

Inhalant-related disorders
- 304.60 Inhalant Dependence
- 305.90 Inhalant Abuse
- 292.89 Inhalant Intoxication
- 292.81 Inhalant Intoxication Delirium
- 292.82 Inhalant-Induced Persisting Dementia
- 292.xx Inhalant-Induced Psychotic Disorder
  where xx is

.11 With Delusions

.12 With Hallucinations

- 292.84 Inhalant-Induced Mood Disorder
- 292.89 Inhalant-Induced Anxiety Disorder
- 292.9 Inhalant-Related Disorder NOS

Nicotine-related disorders

- 305.10 Nicotine Dependence
- 292.0 Nicotine Withdrawal
- 292.9 Nicotine-Related Disorder NOS

Opioid-related disorders

- 304.00 Opioid Dependence
- 305.50 Opioid Abuse
- 292.89 Opioid Intoxication

    Specify if: With Perceptual Disturbances

- 292.0 Opioid Withdrawal
- 292.81 Opioid Intoxication Delirium
- 292.xx Opioid-Induced Psychotic Disorder, where xx is

    .11 With Delusions

    .12 With Hallucinations

- 292.84 Opioid-Induced Mood Disorder
- 292.89 Opioid-Induced Sexual Dysfunction
- 292.89 Opioid-Induced Sleep Disorder
- 292.9 Opioid-Related Disorder NOS

Phencyclidine (or phencyclidine-like)-related disorders

- 304.90 Phencyclidine Dependence
- 305.90 Phencyclidine Abuse
- 292.89 Phencyclidine Intoxication

    Specify if: With Perceptual Disturbances

- 292.81 Phencyclidine Intoxication Delirium
- 292.xx Phencyclidine-Induced Psychotic Disorder, where xx is

    .11 With Delusions

    .12 With Hallucinations

- 292.84 Phencyclidine-Induced Mood Disorder
- 292.89 Phencyclidine-Induced Anxiety Disorder
- 292.9 Phencyclidine-Related Disorder NOS

Sedative-, hypnotic- or anxiolytic-related disorders

- 304.10 Sedative, Hypnotic or Anxiolytic Dependence
- 305.40 Sedative, Hypnotic or Anxiolytic Abuse
- 292.89 Sedative, Hypnotic or Anxiolytic Intoxication
- 292.0 Sedative, Hypnotic or Anxiolytic Withdrawal
    Specify if: With Perceptual Disturbances
- 292.81 Sedative, Hypnotic or Anxiolytic Intoxication Delirium
- 292.81 Sedative, Hypnotic or Anxiolytic Withdrawal Delirium
- 292.82 Sedative-, Hypnotic- or Anxiolytic-Induced Persisting Dementia
- 292.83 Sedative-, Hypnotic- or Anxiolytic-Induced Persisting Amnestic Disorder
- 292.xx Sedative-, Hypnotic- or Anxiolytic-Induced Psychotic Disorder, where xx is
    .11 With Delusions
    .12 With Hallucinations
- 292.84 Sedative-, Hypnotic- or Anxiolytic-Induced Mood Disorder
- 292.89 Sedative-, Hypnotic- or Anxiolytic-Induced Anxiety Disorder
- 292.89 Sedative-, Hypnotic- or Anxiolytic-Induced Sexual Dysfunction
- 292.89 Sedative-, Hypnotic- or Anxiolytic-Induced Sleep Disorder
- 292.9 Sedative-, Hypnotic- or Anxiolytic-Related Disorder NOS

Polysubstance-related disorders
- 304.80 Polysubstance Dependence

Other (or unknown) substance-related disorders
- 304.90 Other (or Unknown) Substance Dependence
- 305.90 Other (or Unknown) Substance Abuse
- 292.89 Other (or Unknown) Substance Intoxication (183)
    Specify if: With Perceptual Disturbances

- 292.0 Other (or Unknown) Substance Withdrawal
    Specify if: With Perceptual Disturbances
- 292.81 Other (or Unknown) Substance-Induced Delirium
- 292.82 Other (or Unknown) Substance-Induced Persisting Dementia
- 292.83 Other (or Unknown) Substance-Induced Persisting Amnestic Disorder
- 292.xx Other (or Unknown) Substance-Induced Psychotic Disorder, where xx is
    .11 With Delusions
    .12 With Hallucinations
- 292.84 Other (or Unknown) Substance-Induced Mood Disorder
- 292.89 Other (or Unknown) Substance-Induced Anxiety Disorder
- 292.89 Other (or Unknown) Substance-Induced Sexual Dysfunction
- 292.89 Other (or Unknown) Substance-Induced Sleep Disorder
- 292.9 Other (or Unknown) Substance-Related Disorder NOS

Schizophrenia and other psychotic disorders
- 295.xx Schizophrenia, where xx is
    .30 Paranoid Type
    .10 Disorganized Type
    .20 Catatonic Type
    .90 Undifferentiated Type
    .60 Residual Type
- 295.40 Schizophreniform Disorder
    Without Good Prognostic Features
    With Good Prognostic Features
- 295.70 Schizoaffective Disorder
    Bipolar Type
    Depressive Type
- 297.1 Delusional Disorder
    Erotomanic Type
    Grandiose Type

  Jealous Type
  Persecutory Type
  Somatic Type
  Mixed Type
  Unspecified Type
- 298.8 Brief Psychotic Disorder
  Specify if: With Marked Stressor(s)/Without
    Marked Stressor(s)/With Postpartum Onset
- 297.3 Shared Psychotic Disorder
- 293.xx Psychotic Disorder Due to. . . [Indicate
  the General Medical Condition]
    .81 With Delusions
    .82 With Hallucinations
- ---.- Substance-Induced Psychotic Disorder (refer
  to Substance-Related Disorders for substance-
  specific codes)
    Specify if: With Onset During Intoxication/
      With Onset During Withdrawal
- 298.9 Psychotic Disorder NOS

Mood disorders
- 296.xx Major Depressive Disorder
    .2x Single Episode
    .3x Recurrent
- 300.4 Dysthymic Disorder
    Specify if: Early Onset/Late Onset
    Specify if: With Atypical Features
- 311 Depressive Disorder NOS
- 296.xx Bipolar I Disorder
    .0x Single Manic Episode
    Specify if: Mixed
    .40 Most Recent Episode Hypomanic
    .4x Most Recent Episode Manic
    .6x Most Recent Episode Mixed
    .5x Most Recent Episode Depressed
    .7 Most Recent Episode Unspecified
- 296.89 Bipolar II Disorder
    Specify (current or most recent episode):
      Hypomanic/Depressed
- 301.13 Cyclothymic Disorder

- 296.80 Bipolar Disorder NOS
- 293.83 Mood Disorder Due to. . .[Indicate the General Medical Condition]
    With Depressive Features
    With Major Depressive-Like Episode
    With Manic Features
    With Mixed Features
- ---.- Substance-Induced Mood Disorder (refer to Substance-Related Disorders for substance-specific codes)
    With Depressive Features
    With Manic Features
    With Mixed Features
Specify if: With Onset During Intoxication/With Onset During Withdrawal
- 296.90 Mood Disorder NOS

Code current state of Major Depressive Disorder or Bipolar I Disorder in fifth digit:
    1 = Mild
    2 = Moderate
    3 = Severe Without Psychotic Features
    4 = Severe With Psychotic Features
    Specify: Mood-Congruent Psychotic Features/ Mood-Incongruent Psychotic Features
    5 = In Partial Remission
    6 = In Full Remission
    0 = Unspecified

Anxiety disorders
- 300.01 Panic Disorder Without Agoraphobia
- 300.21 Panic Disorder With Agoraphobia
- 300.22 Agoraphobia Without History of Panic Disorder
- 300.29 Specific Phobia
    Animal Type
    Natural Environment Type
    Blood-Injection-Injury Type
    Situational Type
    Other Type
- 300.23 Social Phobia

Specify if: Generalized
- 300.3 Obsessive-Compulsive Disorder
    Specify if: With Poor Insight
- 309.81 Post-traumatic Stress Disorder
    Specify if: Acute/Chronic
    Specify if: With Delayed Onset
- 308.3 Acute Stress Disorder
- 300.02 Generalized Anxiety Disorder
- 293.89 Anxiety Disorder Due to. . .[Indicate the
  General Medical Condition]
    Specify if: With Generalized Anxiety/With
        Panic Attacks/With Obsessive-Compulsive
        Symptoms
- ---.- Substance-Induced Anxiety Disorder (refer
  to Substance-Related Disorders for substance-
  specific codes)
    Specify if: With Generalized Anxiety/With
        Panic Attacks/With Obsessive-Compulsive
        Symptoms/With Phobic Symptoms
    Specify if: With Onset During Intoxication/
        With Onset During Withdrawal
- 300.00 Anxiety Disorder NOS

Somatoform disorders
- 300.81 Somatization Disorder
- 300.81 Undifferentiated Somatoform Disorder
- 300.11 Conversion Disorder
    With Motor Symptom or Deficit
    With Sensory Symptom or Deficit
    With Seizures or Convulsions
    With Mixed Presentation
- 307.xx Pain Disorder, where xx is
    .80 Associated With Psychological Factors
    .89 Associated With Both Psychological
        Factors and a General Medical Condition
    Specify if: Acute/Chronic
- 300.7 Hypochondriasis
    Specify if: With Poor Insight
- 300.7 Body Dysmorphic Disorder
- 300.81 Somatoform Disorder NOS

Factitious disorders
- 300.xx Factitious Disorder, where xx is
    - .16 With Predominantly Psychological Signs and Symptoms
    - .19 With Predominantly Physical Signs and Symptoms
    - .19 With Combined Psychological and Physical Signs and Symptoms
- 300.19 Factitious Disorder NOS

Dissociative disorders
- 300.12 Dissociative Amnesia
- 300.13 Dissociative Fugue
- 300.14 Dissociative Identity Disorder
- 300.6 Depersonalization Disorder
- 300.15 Dissociative Disorder NOS

Sexual and gender identity disorders
Sexual dysfunctions
- 302.71 Hypoactive Sexual Desire Disorder
- 302.79 Sexual Aversion Disorder
- 302.72 Female Sexual Arousal Disorder
- 302.72 Male Erectile Disorder
- 302.73 Female Orgasmic Disorder
- 302.74 Male Orgasmic Disorder
- 302.75 Premature Ejaculation
- 302.76 Dyspareunia (Not Due to a General Medical Condition)
- 306.51 Vaginismus (Not Due to a General Medical Condition)
- 625.8 Female Hypoactive Sexual Desire Disorder Due to. . .[indicate the General Medical Condition]
- 608.89 Male Hypoactive Sexual Desire Disorder Due to. . .[Indicate the General Medical Condition]
- 607.84 Male Erectile Disorder Due to. . .[Indicate the General Medical Condition]
- 625.0 Female Dyspareunia Due to. . .[Indicate the General Medical Condition]

- 608.89 Male Dyspareunia Due to. . .[Indicate the General Medical Condition]
- 625.8 Other Female Sexual Dysfunction Due to. . .[Indicate the General Medical Condition]
- 608.89 Other Male Sexual Dysfunction Due to. . .[Indicate the General Medical Condition]
- ---.- Substance-Induced Sexual Dysfunction (refer to Substance-Related Disorders for substance-specific codes)
    Specify if: With Impaired Desire/With Impaired Arousal/With Impaired Orgasm/ With Sexual Pain
    Specify if: With Onset During Intoxication
- 302.70 Sexual Dysfunction NOS

Paraphilias
- 302.4 Exhibitionism
- 302.81 Fetishism
- 302.89 Frotteurism
- 302.2 Pedophilia
    Specify if: Sexually Attracted to Males/ Sexually Attracted to Females/Sexually Attracted to Both
    Specify if: Limited to Incest
    Specify type: Exclusive Type/Non-exclusive Type
- 302.83 Sexual Masochism
- 302.84 Sexual Sadism
- 302.3 Transvestic Fetishism
    Specify if: With Gender Dysphoria
- 302.82 Voyeurism
- 302.9 Paraphilia NOS

Gender identity disorders
- 302.xx Gender Identity Disorder, where x(x) is
    .6 in Children
    .85 in Adolescents or Adults
    Specify if: Sexually Attracted to Males/ Sexually Attracted to Females/Sexually Attracted to Both/Sexually Attracted to Neither

- 302.6 Gender Identity Disorder NOS
- 302.9 Sexual Disorder NOS

Eating disorders
- 307.1 Anorexia Nervosa
    Restricting Type
    Binge-Eating/Purging Type
- 307.51 Bulimia Nervosa
    Purging Type
    Non-purging Type
- 307.50 Eating Disorder NOS

Sleep disorders
Primary sleep disorders – Dyssomnias
- 307.42 Primary Insomnia
- 307.44 Primary Hypersomnia
    Specify if: Recurrent
- 347 Narcolepsy
- 780.59 Breathing-Related Sleep Disorder
- 307.45 Circadian Rhythm Sleep Disorder
    Delayed Sleep Phase Type
    Jet Lag Type
    Shift Work Type
    Unspecified Type
- 307.47 Dyssomnia NOS
Primary sleep disorders – Parasomnias
- 307.47 Nightmare Disorder
- 307.46 Sleep Terror Disorder
- 307.46 Sleepwalking Disorder
- 307.47 Parasomnia NOS
Sleep disorders related to another medical
disorder
- 307.42 Insomnia Related to. . .[Indicate the Axis
  I or Axis II Disorder]
- 307.44 Hypersomnia Related to. . .[Indicate the
  Axis I or Axis II Disorder]
Other sleep disorders
- 780.xx Sleep Disorder Due to. . .[Indicate the
  General Medical Condition]
    .52 Insomnia Type
    .54 Hypersomnia Type

.59 Parasomnia Type

.59 Mixed Type

- ---.- Substance-Induced Sleep Disorder (refer to Substance-Related Disorders for substance-specific codes)

    Insomnia Type

    Hypersomnia Type

    Parasomnia Type

    Mixed Type

    Specify if: With Onset During Intoxication/ With Onset During Withdrawal

Impulse-control disorders not elsewhere classified

- 312.34 Intermittent Explosive Disorder
- 312.32 Kleptomania
- 312.33 Pyromania
- 312.31 Pathological Gambling
- 312.39 Trichotillomania
- 312.30 Impulse-Control Disorder NOS

Adjustment disorders

- 309.xx Adjustment Disorder, where x(x) is

    .0 With Depressed Mood

    .24 With Anxiety

    .28 With Mixed Anxiety and Depressed Mood

    .3 With Disturbance of Conduct

    .4 With Mixed Disturbance of Emotions and Conduct

    .9 Unspecified

    Specify if: Acute/Chronic

Other conditions that may be a focus of clinical attention

Axis II: Personality disorders; mental retardation

Personality disorders

- 301.0 Paranoid Personality Disorder
- 301.20 Schizoid Personality Disorder
- 301.22 Schizotypal Personality Disorder
- 301.7 Antisocial Personality Disorder
- 301.83 Borderline Personality Disorder
- 301.50 Histrionic Personality Disorder
- 301.81 Narcissistic Personality Disorder

- 301.82 Avoidant Personality Disorder
- 301.6 Dependent Personality Disorder
- 301.4 Obsessive-Compulsive Personality Disorder
- 301.9 Personality Disorder NOS

Mental retardation
- 317 Mild Mental Retardation
- 318.0 Moderate Mental Retardation
- 318.1 Severe Mental Retardation
- 318.2 Profound Mental Retardation
- 319 Mental Retardation, Severity Unspecified

Axis III: General medical conditions

Infectious and parasitic diseases
Neoplasms
Endocrine, nutritional and metabolic diseases and immunity disorders
Diseases of the blood and blood-forming organs
Diseases of the nervous system and sense organs
Diseases of the circulatory system
Diseases of the respiratory system
Diseases of the digestive system
Diseases of the genito-urinary system
Complications of pregnancy, childbirth and the puerperium
Diseases of the skin and subcutaneous tissue
Diseases of the musculoskeletal system and connective tissue
Congenital anomalies
Certain conditions originating in the perinatal period
Symptoms, signs and ill-defined conditions
Injury and poisoning

Axis IV: Psychosocial and environmental problems

Problems with primary support group
Problems related to the social environment
Educational problems
Occupational problems
Housing problems
Economic problems

Problems with access to health care services
Problems related to interaction with the legal
  system/crime
Other psychosocial and environmental problems

Axis V: Global assessment of functioning

14

THE PSYCHIATRIC WARD ROUND AND THE MULTIDISCIPLINARY (MULTIPROFESSIONAL) TEAM

In order to focus on ward rounds it is important to look at the functioning of professionals in psychiatry in relation to the patient.

Over the last 100 years in psychiatry ideas have continued to be revisited and previous experience has been temporarily forgotten. The treatment of the socially disadvantaged mentally ill shows cyclical patterns of enthusiastic optimism alternating with pessimism and lack of realism. When this fails to move forward, it is easy to blame society, government or an obsolete system such as care in the community. Psychiatry has been politicized and it is easy to become service oriented rather than looking at both the needs of patients and the risk to them as we follow the latest fashionable theme.

Psychiatry has moved out of the asylum and into the general hospital and medical school. The ward round has similarly been adopted, although is not usually conducted in the same way as a medical ward round.

The purpose of the ward round is to review the state of the patient at that moment and to formulate and adopt a future care plan. It also has a role in bringing all the professionals involved with the patient together.

It can be a frightening experience for a patient to attend a ward round where key sensitive issues concerning him or her are being debated. Some ward rounds do not have patients attending and are mostly management oriented. In such cases the opportunity is made available for the patients to discuss their treatment and progress either before or after the ward round. However, many patients appreciate the chance to 'argue their corner' during the ward round.

The setting of the ward round should be comfortable, and the usual format is to arrange the chairs in a circle. Most professionals have to keep written records of the proceedings, although with the growing trend towards multiprofessional notes this will not always be necessary. If needed, translators should be arranged beforehand for those patients who require them.

When the patient attends he or she should be made to feel welcome and at ease and not be asked insensitive questions about topics such as his or her sex life in front of everyone else. The discussion should be enabling rather than confrontational, and every effort should be made to reach an amicable conclusion with a care plan that is safe and acceptable to everyone. If refreshment is being offered, it should be offered to the patient as well. For the sake of all those involved the ward round should not last longer than 4 hours.

The patient is not the only point of conflict in the ward round. Interactions between various members of the multiprofessional team can also lead to interpersonal friction. A ward round will include several disciplines, including occupational therapists, nurses, doctors and social workers. In addition there may be pharmacists, various professional visitors, and sometimes relatives.

The various professionals view the patient's needs and problems differently, although often with considerable overlap. This can be and usually is enabling, but occasionally two differing points of view may cause conflict, e.g. a sociological approach may be incompatible with a biological approach. The resolution of such a problem depends upon mutual respect and, to some extent, on the skill and tact of the other people present. The various professionals will usually have differing levels of experience, and people with widely differing abilities may be present. A second-year occupational therapist may, for example, find it difficult to work closely with a very experienced ward manager, or vice versa. The personalities of all those present may or may not promote smooth working relationships. The chairperson will be expected to iron out these wrinkles, and for this reason he or she should be skilled and experienced. Sometimes there will be a rotating chairperson, while in other teams it will always be the same person, but it does not always have to be the consultant of the team.

Adequate preparation for the ward round can allow it to run more smoothly. The patient's files which are going to be discussed should be assembled in the correct order beside the person whose duty it is to write in them, e.g. the junior doctor writes in the medical files and the nurse writes in the nursing file, etc.

A written summary of patients to be discussed, with the relevant information attached, can be helpful. This information can include the date of admission, mental health status and progress. Sufficient tea, coffee and biscuits will help to keep the group focused, hard-working and happy.

Presenting cases

The headings under which a case should be presented in a psychiatric ward round include the following.

Psychiatric history

List the following:

- reason for referral, complaints, history of the presenting illness;
- family history;

- family psychiatric history;
- personal history;
- past medical history;
- past psychiatric history;
- psychoactive substance use;
- forensic history;
- premorbid personality.

Mental State Examination
List the following:
- appearance and behaviour;
- speech;
- mood;
- thought content;
- abnormal beliefs and interpretations of events;
- abnormal experiences;
- cognitive state;
- insight.

Physical examination
Investigations
- further information;
- first-line investigations;
- second-line investigations.

Diagnosis or differential diagnosis
This can be followed by a description of the management thus far.

15

KEEPING WARD CASE-NOTES

Case-notes are the form in which information is collected and stored. The information usually comes from a variety of sources, including doctors, nurses, occupational therapists, psychologists, etc. Each hospital may have its own case-notes, and these are the responsibility of the medical records department and not the property of the patient. This means that if a patient is routinely admitted to two different hospitals he or she will have two sets of notes and the patient will have to give the respective medical records departments permission – as will the doctors in charge of the patient – to read what is in the set of notes at the other hospital.

Medical case-notes used to be the property of the doctor who made the record, but this is now only the case in some private hospitals.

Case-notes are not just intended to aid the clinician's memory, but are an essential source of information for the future. There is usually a recognized format for case-notes, and the various colleges suggest the material which should be covered. The case-notes are also important from a medico-legal point of view, and as such need to be clearly legible, dated and signed, and should not be altered once written, unless it is necessary to correct factual inaccuracies, in which case the entry should again be dated and signed.

The case-notes may be called upon in the event of an inquest, trial or complaint by the patient. The patient is also entitled to have access to his or her notes, so it is a good idea to write in patient-sensitive language. The case record does not have to be stored in paper form, but may be kept on a computer or held by the patient in note form (e.g. as in obstetric records) or as a smart card.

The admission note

When a patient is admitted to hospital urgently, as is the case for most psychiatric patients, the admitting doctor will have only limited time and may not be involved with the patient in the future. The record should include the following:

- reason for admission;
- any information about decisions for immediate treatment;
- Mental State Examination on admission;
- information from an informant if available;
- systematic history, if there is time;
- physical examination, if possible;
- provisional plan of management agreed with senior nurses on duty at the time;
- any treatment administered at the time of admission.

Progress notes – day-to-day notes

Progress notes will be of little value when case-notes are reviewed if they are not written thoughtfully. The notes should state in what way the patient feels better or worse, e.g. 'is no longer restless and was able to sit through the interview'.

Treatment should also be recorded in the progress notes, even though it is also written on the prescription card.

A regular Mental State Examination should be recorded, together with any other forms of treatment such as cognitive therapy or electroconvulsive therapy (ECT).

Ward-round notes

A careful note of decisions reached during the ward round and at other meetings should be kept. The record should be dated, signed and marked 'ward round'. If the patient is interviewed, a record of the interview – either verbatim or summarized – will be useful and of particular importance in devising the care and discharge plans.

Multidisciplinary notes and integrated care plans
Historically, members of various disciplines looking after the psychiatric in-patient have kept their own case-files on each patient – resulting, for example, in psychiatric case-notes, social work case-notes, and so on. There is of necessity a great deal of overlap in the information which each discipline keeps, and such duplication is probably unnecessary. An increasing trend is to have multidisciplinary notes with a unitary care plan. There are two alternative ways in which members of various disciplines contribute to such multidisciplinary case-notes. One possibility is that each member of staff writing about the patient does so in the case-notes straight after the previous entry (possibly by a member of a different discipline) so that the result is a sequential set of notes with signed contributions from different disciplines. The alternative is that the set of case-notes is divided into different sections – one or more for each discipline. This causes problems with access to notes being more difficult, and conflict arises over responsibilities for maintaining the file and adding the necessary information. There are also problems with regard to the number of sections/compartments in the file and their organization.

Most files include the following:
• demographic details such as name, sex, age, address, etc.;
• problems identified;
• care plan;
• progress notes;
• correspondence;
• Mental Health Act legislation;
• investigations.

Integrated care plans

In this case the format is similar to that in multi-disciplinary notes, with standards which have been agreed by the team being implemented, and variance tracking is also built into the case-notes so that standards can be improved and self-audit can take place.

Part II

Treatment

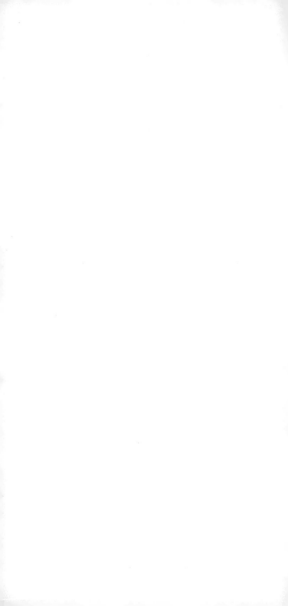

16

PSYCHOTHERAPIES

COGNITIVE BEHAVIOUR THERAPY

Cognitive behaviour therapy is an individual short-term structured psychotherapy in which the therapist collaborates with the patient to achieve alteration of the unhelpful thoughts or behaviours that are causing the problem. It can be used either in conjunction with medication, or on its own.

The two components are as follows.

- Cognitive therapy – the therapist works with the patient to look at the current problem and how to resolve it using Aaron Beck's ideas. Cognitive therapy utilizes the concept that 'an individual's affect and behaviour are largely determined by the way in which he or she structures the world'.
- Behaviour therapy – behaviour techniques naturally complement cognitive techniques, and their purpose is to help the patient to understand the inaccuracy of his or her cognitive assumptions and to learn new ways of dealing with the problem.

Treatment strategies

Patient selection is important, as someone who cannot accept the model would not benefit from therapy based on it. Usually therapy is of short duration, typically 12–20 weekly sessions of 1 hour. Maintenance can occur over a longer period.

The therapist needs to understand the life experience of each patient, and the approach is problem oriented rather than focusing on the origins of the problem. The therapist's first approach is educational, explaining about assumptions or schemas based on early experiences, and how they cause us to think in a certain way about ourselves, the world in which we live and the future. Schemas can be helpful, but they can also be a hindrance, and are called 'dysfunctional schemas'. They can be rigid, extreme, resistant to alteration, and negative.

The therapist and patient work together as a team, formulating hypotheses and using them during the course of the therapy. The cognitive aspects use four processes:

- eliciting negative automatic thoughts or cognitive distortions, e.g. when faced with a new experience an automatic thought is 'I will never be able to do this';
- the therapist helps the patient to test the validity of these thoughts and to work out alternative explanations;
- the therapist and the patient identify maladaptive assumptions;
- faulty logic is exposed.

Each session should have an agenda. The patient works on the problem at home, not just in the therapy session. There is feedback to the patient about change, and strategies are reviewed.

Cognitive behaviour therapy is effective in the treatment of:

- depression;
- panic and anxiety;
- obsessive-compulsive disorder;
- phobias.

It is also used in the treatment of hypochrondiasis and post-traumatic stress disorder.

INDIVIDUAL PSYCHOTHERAPY

Individual long-term psychodynamic psychotherapy takes place within the framework of the therapist's school of psychotherapy, e.g. Freudian, Jungian or

Kleinian. It may take place over a long period, e.g. five (Monday to Friday) 50-minute sessions over several years. The most important elements of the therapy include:

- free association;
- dream analysis;
- analysis of the transference;
- analysis of the countertransference;
- working with the patient's resistance and defence mechanisms;
- using clarification, linking, reflection, interpretation and confrontation.

Its main aims are:

- symptom relief;
- personality change.

Disorders in which individual psychotherapy may be helpful include:

- anxiety disorders;
- hysterical conversion disorders;
- obsessive-compulsive disorder;
- psychosomatic disorders.

In general, individual psychotherapy is unsuitable for patients suffering from acute psychotic disorders.

Brief focal psychotherapy

This is much shorter and more focused than individual long-term psychotherapy.

Group psychotherapy

This has similar aims to individual psychotherapy, but is carried out with a group of patients and one therapist.

Family therapy

In this form of group psychotherapy the group consists of members of one family, together with usually either one therapist or two co-therapists.

Marital therapy

Marital therapy can utilize behavioural models and contracts, and is offered to couples needing help to resolve relationship difficulties.

Sex therapy

Sex therapy can be used to treat couples with sexual dysfunction. It can utilize behavioural techniques and psychotherapeutic techniques.

Art therapy and music therapy

These therapies are essentially non-verbal forms of psychotherapy, that can be administered individually or in groups, in which the patient communicates with the therapist by means of art or music. Such therapies can be usefully employed in cases in which it is difficult for the patient to communicate verbally, e.g. children, those with severe learning difficulties, and those with brain damage. As with forms of psychotherapy based on speech, the therapist fosters an environment in which the patient can free-associate, in the form of his or her artistic or muscial expression. Occasionally special techniques are used to encourage this, e.g. a right-handed patient may be asked to paint with his or her left hand. The resulting art or music may be considered to include a manifestation of the unconscious, and can be interpreted accordingly by the therapist.

17

PSYCHOTROPIC MEDICATION

This section is meant to provide only an outline of the different types of psychotropic medication available. The guidelines provided by the most recent formularies (the British National Formulary in the UK) and the manufacturers should always be referred to and followed. Note also that the examples given for each class of drug are not meant to be exhaustive.

ANTIPSYCHOTICS (NEUROLEPTICS)

Atypical antipsychotics are less likely to cause movement disorders than are the older typical antipsychotics. However, at the time of writing atypical antipsychotics are more expensive than typical antipsychotics, and they are not available in the form of depot preparations.

TYPICAL ANTIPSYCHOTICS

In the following classification, note that the piperidine group of phenothiazines includes thioridazine, which is classed here as an atypical antipsychotic.

1. phenothiazines – aliphatic
   - chlorpromazine
   - methotrimeprazine
   - promazine
2. phenothiazines – piperazines
   - fluphenazine
   - trifluoperazine

- perphenazine
- prochlorperazine
3. phenothiazines – piperidines
   - pipothiazine palmitate
   - pericyazine
4. butyrophenones
   - haloperidol
   - droperidol
   - benperidol
   - trifluperidol
5. thioxanthenes
   - flupenthixol
   - zuclopenthixol
6. diphenylbutyl-piperidines
   - pimozide
   - fluspirilene
7. loxapine

The movement disorders that may result from treatment with typical antipsychotics include:
- akathisia – this may develop within the first 2 days of treatment;
- dystonias – acute dystonias may develop within the first day of treatment, while chronic dystonias may take months or years to develop;
- Parkinsonism – this may be seen within weeks of treatment;
- tardive dyskinesia – this usually takes months or years to develop, and may not be reversible.
   Other important side-effects include:
- cardiac arrhythmias – these are particularly important in the cases of pimozide and thioridazine; in the UK the Committee on Safety of Medicines recommends that a baseline ECG should be carried out before commencing treatment with pimozide, and periodic ECGs thereafter;
- peripheral antimuscarinic actions – such as dry mouth, blurred vision, urinary retention, constipation, nasal congestion;

- central antimuscarinic actions – such as convulsions and pyrexia;
- hyperprolactinaemia – which may result in galactorrhoea, gynaecomastia, menstrual disturbances;
- reduced sperm count, reduced libido;
- antiadrenergic actions – such as postural hypotension and ejaculatory failure;
- drowsiness;
- neuroleptic malignant syndrome – this is rare but potentially fatal; it is characterized by hyperthermia, fluctuating consciousness level, and autonomic dysfunction (pallor, sweating, tachycardia, labile blood pressure, urinary incontinence).

ATYPICAL ANTIPSYCHOTICS

The atypical antipsychotics include:

- clozapine;
- risperidone;
- sulpiride (a substituted benzamide);
- thioridazine;
- olanzapine;
- sertindole;
- zotepine (being tested at the time of writing);
- amperozide (being tested at the time of writing).
- quetiapine
- amisulpride (a benzamide)

A baseline ECG should be carried out before commencing treatment with sertindole, and periodic ECGs thereafter. However, sertindole, which exhibits limbic selectivity (selectivity for dopaminergic neurones in the ventral tegmental area rather than the pars compacta of the substantia nigra) does not appear to be more cardiotoxic than most other atypical antipsychotics.

Clozapine

Contraindications

These include:

- severe cardiac disease;
- history of drug-induced neutropenia/agranu-
  locytosis;
- bone marrow disorders;
- alcoholic and toxic psychoses;
- history of circulatory collapse or paralytic ileus;
- drug intoxication;
- coma;
- severe central nervous system depression;
- uncontrolled epilepsy;
- pregnancy;
- breast-feeding.

Side-effects

These include:

- many of the same side-effects as chlorpromazine,
  except that it causes decreased sedation, increased antimuscarinic symptoms and decreased
  extrapyramidal symptoms;
- neutropenia and potentially fatal agranulocytosis,
  hence the need for regular haematological monitoring (see below);
- pyrexia (but exclude an infection or agranulocytosis);
- headache and dizziness;
- hypersalivation;
- urinary incontinence;
- priapism;
- pericarditis and myocarditis;
- delirium;
- hypotension – rarely circulatory collapse with
  cardiac and respiratory arrest;
- nausea and vomiting;
- hyperglycaemia.

Haematological monitoring

Owing to the side-effect of neutropenia and potentially fatal agranulocytosis, in the UK the initiation

of treatment with clozapine must be in hospital in-patients, with the patient being registered with the Clozaril Patient Monitoring Service (CPMS). The CPMS provides for the required leucocyte counts as well as a drug supply audit to ensure that clozapine is withdrawn from any patient with an abnormal leucocyte count. In the UK, details of the CPMS can be obtained from:

The Clozaril Patient Monitoring Service Manager
Novartis Pharmaceuticals UK Ltd
Frimley Business Park
Frimley
Camberley
Surrey GU16 5SG

Tel: 01276 692255
Fax: 01276 692508

At the time of writing, in order to initiate treatment with clozapine in the UK, the following criteria should be fulfilled:
• the patient is a hospital in-patient;
• the patient is registered with the CPMS;
• the white blood cell count $> 3.5 \times 10^9$ L^{-1};
• the differential blood count is normal.

It is generally recommended that clozapine should not be given in combination with typical antipsychotics (including depot preparations), which may have a myelosuppressive action. During treatment with clozapine the white blood count and differential count must be monitored weekly for the first 18 weeks, and at least at 2-week intervals for the first year of treatment. After the patient has been on treatment for 1 year, with stable neutrophil counts over that period, then the frequency of monitoring may be changed to 4-week intervals. Monitoring must continue for as long as the patient is being treated with clozapine. GPs can now pre-scribe clozapine if the patient is stabilized and the drug is being prescribed every 4 weeks.

ANTIPSYCHOTIC DEPOT PREPARATIONS

Contraindications
These include:
- childhood;
- confusional states;
- coma caused by central nervous system depressants;
- Parkinsonism;
- intolerance to antipsychotics;
- Lewy body dementia.

Side-effects
In addition to the side-effects of the antipsychotic itself, the following side-effects may occur at the injection site as a result of depot injections:
- pain;
- erythema;
- swelling;
- nodule formation.

Administration
The British National Formulary (BNF) notes the following points concerning the administering of antipsychotic depot injections:

Depot antipsychotics are administered by deep intramuscular injection at intervals of 1 to 4 weeks. Patients should first be given a small test dose as undesirable side-effects are prolonged. In general, not more than 2–3 mL of oily injection should be administered at any one site; correct injection technique (including the use of z-track technique) and rotation of injection sites are essential. If the dose needs to be reduced to alleviate side-effects it is important to recognize that the plasma level may not fall for some time after reducing the dose, therefore it may be a month or longer before side-effects subside.

ANTIPSYCHOTIC DOSES ABOVE THE BNF UPPER LIMIT

The Royal College of Psychiatrists has published advice on the use of antipsychotic doses above the

BNF upper limit. This advice is reproduced in the BNF:

Unless otherwise stated, doses in the BNF are licensed doses — any higher dose is therefore *unlicensed.*

1. Consider alternative approaches including adjuvant therapy and newer or atypical neuroleptics such as clozapine.

2. Bear in mind risk factors, including obesity — particular caution is indicated in older patients, especially those over 70 years.

3. Consider the potential for drug interactions (published in an appendix to the BNF).

4. Carry out ECG to exclude untoward abnormalities such as prolonged QT interval; repeat ECG periodically, and reduce the dose if a prolonged QT interval or other adverse abnormality develops.

5. Increase the dose slowly and not more often than once weekly.

6. Carry out regular pulse, blood pressure and temperature checks; ensure that the patient maintains an adequate fluid intake.

7. Consider high-dose therapy to be for a limited period only and review it regularly; abandon it if there is no improvement after 3 months (return to standard dosage).

Important. When prescribing an antipsychotic for administration on an emergency basis, it must be borne in mind that the intramuscular dose should be *lower* than the corresponding oral dose (owing to the absence of a first-pass effect), particularly if the patient is very active (increased blood flow to muscle considerably increases the rate of absorption). The prescription should specify the dose in the context of *each route* and should *not* imply that the same dose can be given by mouth or by intramuscular injection. The dose should be reviewed *daily.*

ANTIMUSCARINIC DRUGS USED IN PARKINSONISM

These include:
- procyclidine
- benzhexol
- benztropine
- orphenadrine
- biperiden
- methixene

Contraindications
These include:
- untreated urinary retention;
- closed-angle glaucoma;
- gastrointestinal obstruction.

Side-effects
These include:
- dry mouth;
- gastrointestinal disturbances;
- dizziness;
- blurred vision;
- urinary retention;
- tachycardia;
- hypersensitivity;
- nervousness;
- mental confusion, excitement, psychiatric disturbance – with high doses in susceptible patients;
- may worsen tardive dyskinesia.

Use
These drugs should not be prescribed routinely to patients being treated with typical antipsychotics, but only if and when such patients develop Parkinsonism. This is because:
- not all such patients develop Parkinsonism;
- these drugs have side-effects, as described above.

LITHIUM

Lithium salts (particularly lithium carbonate and lithium citrate) are used in:
- prophylaxis of biopolar mood disorder;
- treatment of mania/hypomania;
- treatment of resistant depression;
- prophylaxis of recurrent depression;
- treatment of agression;
- treatment of self-mutilation.

Contraindications

These include:

- renal impairment;
- cardiac disease;
- Addison's disease and other conditions with sodium imbalance;
- untreated hypothyroidism.

Side-effects

These include:

- fatigue;
- drowsiness;
- dry mouth;
- a metallic taste;
- polydipsia;
- polyuria;
- nausea;
- vomiting;
- weight gain;
- diarrhoea;
- fine tremor;
- muscle weakness;
- oedema.

Oedema should not be treated with diuretics, since thiazide and loop diuretics reduce lithium excretion and can thereby cause lithium intoxication.

Intoxication

Signs of lithium intoxication include:

- mild drowsiness and sluggishness leading to giddiness and ataxia;
- lack of co-ordination;
- blurred vision;
- tinnitus;
- anorexia;
- dysarthria;
- vomiting;
- diarrhoea;
- coarse tremor;
- muscle weakness.

Severe overdosage

At lithium plasma levels higher than 2 mmol L^{-1} the following effects can occur:

- hyper-reflexia and hyperextension of the limbs;
- toxic psychoses;
- convulsions;
- syncope;
- oliguria;
- circulatory failure;
- coma;
- death.

Chronic therapy

Long-term treatment with lithium may give rise to:

- thyroid function disturbances (goitre, hypo-thyroidism);
- memory impairment;
- nephrotoxicity;
- cardiovascular changes (T-wave flattening on the ECG, arrhythmias).

CARBAMAZEPINE

Carbamazepine is used instead of, or in combination with, lithium in:

- biopolar mood disorder resistant to lithium;
- resistant mania;
- resistant depression.

It is also used in treating epilepsy and the paroxysmal pain of trigeminal neuralgia.

Contraindications

These include:

- atrioventricular (AV) conduction abnormalities (unless paced);
- history of bone marrow depression;
- porphyria.

Side-effects

The main side-effects of carbamazepine include:

- nausea and vomiting;
- dizziness;

- drowsiness;
- headache;
- ataxia;
- confusion and agitation in the elderly;
- visual disturbances, especially double vision (may be associated with peak plasma concentrations);
- constipation or diarrhoea;
- anorexia;
- mild transient generalized erythematous rash;
- blood disorders (leucopenia, thrombocytopenia, agranulocytosis, aplastic anaemia).

ANTIDEPRESSANTS

TRICYCLIC ANTIDEPRESSANTS

Tricyclic antidepressants include:
1. dibenzocycloheptanes:
   - amitriptyline;
   - butriptyline;
   - nortriptyline;
   - protriptyline;
2. iminodibenzyls:
   - clomipramine;
   - desipramine;
   - imipramine;
   - trimipramine;
3. others:
   - dothiepin;
   - doxepin;
   - iprindole;
   - lofepramine.

Of these tricyclic antidepressants, imipramine, for example, is less sedating, amitriptyline is more sedating, and lofepramine is relatively less toxic.

Contraindications
These include:
- recent myocardial infarction;
- arrhythmias – particularly heart block;
- mania;

- severe liver disease.

Side-effects

These include:

1. antimuscarinic symptoms:
   - dry mouth;
   - blurred vision;
   - urinary retention;
   - constipation;
   - drowsiness;
2. antihistaminergic symptoms:
   - weight gain;
   - drowsiness;
3. antiadrenergic symptoms:
   - drowsiness;
   - postural hypotension;
   - sexual dysfunction;
   - cognitive impairment;
4. antiserotonergic symptoms:
   - weight gain;
5. effects of membrane stabilization:
   - cardiotoxicity;
   - decreased seizure threshold;
6. cardiovascular side-effects:
   - ECG changes;
   - arrhythmias;
   - postural hypotension;
   - tachycardia;
   - syncope;
7. allergic and haematological reactions:
   - agranulocytosis;
   - leucopenia;
   - eosinophilia;
   - thrombocytopenia;
   - skin rash;
   - photosensitization;
   - facial oedema;
   - allergic cholestatic jaundice;
8. endocrine side-effects:
   - testicular enlargement;

- gynaecomastia;
- galactorrhoea;
9. tremor;
10. black tongue;
11. paralytic ileus;
12. sweating;
13. hyponatraemia – particularly in the elderly;
14. neuroleptic malignant syndrome (very rare);
15. abnormal liver function tests;
16. movement disorders;
17. pyrexia;
18. (hypo)mania;
19. blood glucose changes.

SELECTIVE SEROTONIN REUPTAKE INHIBITORS (SSRIs)

Selective serotonin reuptake inhibitors include:
- fluvoxamine;
- fluoxetine;
- sertraline;
- paroxetine;
- citalopram;
- nefazodone.

Contraindications
These include:
- mania;
- dehydration.

Side-effects
The more common side-effects include:
- dose-related gastrointestinal side-effects (nausea, vomiting, diarrhoea);
- headache;
- restlessness;
- sleep disturbance;
- anxiety;
- delayed or absent orgasm;
- hyponatraemia.

MONOAMINE OXIDASE INHIBITORS (MAOIs)

Monoamine oxidase inhibitors include:

1. hydrazine compounds:
   - phenelzine;
   - isocarboxazid;
2. non-hydrazine compounds:
   - tranylcypromine.

Contraindications
These include:
- mania;
- hepatic impairment or abnormal liver function tests;
- cerebrovascular disease;
- phaeochromocytoma.

Dangerous food interactions
The inhibition of peripheral pressor amines, particularly dietary tyramine, by MAOIs can lead to a hypertensive crisis when foodstuffs rich in tyramine are eaten. Foods that should be avoided while the patient is being treated with MAOIs include:
- cheese – except cottage cheese and cream cheese;
- meat extracts and yeast extracts;
- alcohol – particularly chianti, fortified wines and beer;
- non-fresh fish;
- non-fresh meat;
- non-fresh poultry;
- offal;
- avocado;
- banana skins;
- broad-bean pods;
- caviar;
- herring – pickled or smoked.

Dangerous drug interactions
Medicines that should be avoided while being treated with MAOIs include:

1. indirectly acting sympathomimetic amines, such as:
   - amphetamine;
   - fenfluramine;
   - ephedrine;
   - phenylpropanolamine;
2. cough mixtures containing sympathomimetics;
3. nasal decongestants containing sympathomimetics;
4. L-dopa;
5. pethidine;
6. tricyclic antidepressants.

Other side-effects
These include:
- antimuscarinic actions;
- hepatotoxicity;
- appetite stimulation;
- weight gain;
- tranylcypromine may cause dependency.

REVERSIBLE INHIBITORS OF MONOAMINE OXIDASE A (RIMAs)

Reversible inhibitors of monoamine oxidase A include:
- moclobemide.

At the time of writing, the following RIMAs are being tested:
- brofaromine;
- cimoxatone;
- toloxatone.

SEROTONIN NORADRENALINE REUPTAKE INHIBITORS (SNRIs)

At the time of writing there is one serotonin noradrenaline reuptake inhibitor (SNRI) in clinical use
- venlafaxine.

The following effects can occur in severe over-dosage:

- arrhythmias;
- convulsions;
- respiratory failure;
- coma;
- death.

NORADRENERGIC AND SPECIFIC SEROTONERGIC ANTIDEPRESSANTS (NaSSAs)

At the time of writing there is one noradrenergic and specific serotonergic antidepressant (NaSSA) in clinical use:

- mirtazapine.

ANXIOLYTICS

BENZODIAZEPINES

Long-acting benzodiazepines include:

- alprazolam;
- bromazepam;
- chlordiazepoxide;
- clobazam;
- clorazepate;
- diazepam;
- flunitrazepam;
- flurazepam;
- medazepam;
- nitrazepam.
  Short-acting benzodiazepines include:
- loprazolam;
- lorazepam;
- lormetazepam;
- oxazepam;
- temazepam.

Contraindications
These include:

- respiratory depression;

- acute pulmonary insufficiency;
- severe hepatic impairment;
- myasthenia gravis;
- sleep apnoea syndrome.

Side-effects

These include:

- drowsiness and lightheadedness the following day;
- confusion and ataxia – particularly in the elderly;
- amnesia;
- dependence;
- paradoxical increase in aggression.

Guidelines on prescribing benzodiazepines

In the UK, the Committee on Safety of Medicines has issued the following advice with respect to the prescription of benzodiazepines.

1. Benzodiazepines are indicated for the short-term relief (2 to 4 weeks only) of anxiety that is severe, disabling or subjecting the individual to unacceptable distress, occurring alone or in association with insomnia or short-term psychosomatic, organic or psychotic illness.
2. The use of benzodiazepines to treat short-term 'mild' anxiety is inappropriate and unsuitable.
3. Benzodiazepines should be used to treat insomnia only when it is severe, disabling or subjecting the individual to extreme distress.

BUSPIRONE

Buspirone is a non-benzodiazepine (an azaspiro-decanedione) anxiolytic in clinical use.

Contraindications

These include:

- epilepsy;
- severe hepatic impairment;
- severe renal impairment;
- pregnancy;

- breast-feeding.

Side-effects
The main side-effects are:
- dizziness;
- headache;
- excitement;
- nausea.

OTHER ANXIOLYTICS

Non-benzodiazepine anxiolytics in clinical use include:
- azaspirodecanediones – buspirone (see above);
- β-adrenoceptor-blocking drugs – e.g. propranolol.

DRUGS USED IN ALCOHOL DEPENDENCE

The following drugs are used in alcohol dependence:
- benzodiazepines (see above);
- chlormethiazole;
- disulfiram;
- acamprosate.

DRUGS USED IN OPIOID DEPENDENCE

The following drugs are used in opioid dependence:
- methadone;
- lofexidine;
- naltrexone.

CYPROTERONE ACETATE

Cyproterone acetate is an antiandrogen used clinically.

Contraindications
These include:
- hepatic disease;
- severe diabetes mellitus (with vascular changes);

- sickle-cell anaemia;
- malignant or wasting disease;
- severe depression;
- history of thromboembolic disorders;
- age < 18 years.

Side-effects

Side-effects in males include:

- inhibition of spermatogenesis;
- tiredness;
- gynaecomastia;
- weight gain;
- improvement of existing acne vulgaris;
- increased scalp hair growth;
- female pattern of pubic hair growth;
- dyspnoea – from high-dose treatment.

THE USE OF DONEPEZIL IN ALZHEIMER'S DISEASE

The acetylcholinesterase inhibitor donepezil, which enhances cholinergic neurotransmission by increasing available acetylcholine at central cholinergic synapses, was licensed for use in the UK in 1997 (Aricept®) for the symptomatic treatment of mild to moderately severe Alzheimer's disease. At the time of writing only one randomized, double-blind, placebo-controlled trial of this drug in Alzheimer's disease has been published (Rogers *et al.* 1996: The efficacy and safety of donepezil in patients with Alzheimer's disease. Results of a US multicentre, randomized, double-blind, placebo-controlled trial. *Dementia* **7**, 293–303). On the basis of this paper, the *Drug and Therapeutics Bulletin* concluded:

In a 12-week, double-blind, placebo-controlled study, donepezil (5 mg daily) improved cognitive function in patients with mild to moderately severe Alzheimer's disease. However, the drug failed to influence day-to-day functioning, quality-of-life measures and rating scores of overall dementia. The clinical significance of the changes for patients and their families or carers is, therefore, unclear. On the published evidence available we cannot recommend the use of donepezil. The position would change if more tangible evidence became available showing that the product offers real improvement in patients' well-being.

(*Drug and Therapeutics Bulletin* **35**, 75–6)

OPTIMIZING PATIENT COMPLIANCE

Factors that can help to optimize patient compliance include:
- patient education;
- setting reasonable expectations;
- reducing the number of tablets to be taken;
- reducing the dosage frequency;
- labelling medicine containers clearly;
- parenteral/depot administration;
- using alternative medication if there are troublesome side-effects;
- involving family members.

It is important to avoid polypharmacy if possible, and to prescribe a simple, straightforward drug regime for elderly patients. Containers used by the elderly should take into account the possibility that the patient may have arthritis, and may also be designed to allow the pharmacist to place the appropriate medication for each intake in clearly labelled boxes.

18

ELECTROCONVULSIVE THERAPY

Electroconvulsive therapy (ECT) is a procedure whereby a small amount of electrical current is sent to the brain, producing a seizure. The patient is anaesthetized and given a muscle relaxant before the current is administered.

It has been proved by double-blind clinical comparisons of bilateral real and simulated ECT to be of clear therapeutic benefit in depressive disorders. It is also used in the treatment of mania and acute catatonic states, to good effect.

Consent to ECT

People with a psychiatric disorder can and should give valid consent to treatment with ECT, even if they have been admitted to hospital against their wishes. The treatment should be adequately explained to the prospective patient by means of both verbal and written material. Some patients by virtue of their mental illness will not be able to give consent, e.g. a very suicidal person or someone who is mute. Informed consent is required before treatment can be given unless statute law or common law provides the consent. If this is the case the treatment should be:

- in the best interest of the person to be treated – to save life or to prevent further deterioration in his or her physical or mental health;
- administered in the manner of best practice of the time as described by a responsible body of medical opinion skilled in the treatment.

Consent should be freely given after adequate explanation of the treatment, the reasons for the treatment, and the procedure, side-effects and alternatives. The patient must also understand that his or her consent can be withdrawn at any time. He or she should not feel under any obligation to consent to treatment.

The ability to give informed consent is a matter of clinical judgement.

Patients presenting for a course of ECT may include:

- an informal patient who has signed a consent form giving valid consent;
- an informal patient who is unable to consent and who requires emergency treatment;
- a detained patient under section who is capable of giving informed consent and has signed a consent form;
- a detained patient under section who does not consent, so that a second opinion needs to be obtained from the Mental Health Act Commission;
- a detained patient under section who is unable to give informed consent, so that a second opinion must be sought;
- a detained patient who requires emergency treatment.

Preparation of patients for ECT

Assessment
- A thorough medical history and physical examination are necessary, noting especially any cardiovascular problems and respiratory problems. A note should be made of dentition, and any hazards pointed out to the anaesthetist.
- Current medication should be scrutinized and any previous anaesthetic problems noted.
- Benzodiazepines are likely to reduce the ability to produce a seizure and, where possible, should not be administered during ECT.

- Tricyclic antidepressants have been associated with seizures and have detrimental effects on cardiac function. They should not be administered to patients with epilepsy or cardiac problems.
- Selective serotonin reuptake inhibitors appear to cause seizures in overdose, but little is known about their effect on seizure threshold in ECT, and prolonged fits have been reported anecdotally. This suggests that treatment should start with a low treatment stimulus (50 mC).
- Anticonvulsants alter the seizure threshold and shorten the duration of the seizure, and may require a high treatment stimulus. Anticonvulsants that are being used for mood stabilization, such as carbamazepine, should be continued during treatment.
- Neuroleptics can reduce the seizure threshold, but this effect is dose dependent.

Investigations
- All patients should have a full blood count and urea and electrolytes determination. An electrocardiogram (ECG) is needed for patients with symptoms of cardiovascular disease.
- Physical illnesses e.g. diabetes, dehydration and hypertension, should be controlled before ECT.
- Afro-Caribbean, Middle Eastern, Asian and Eastern Mediterranean patients must be sickle-cell tested.
- Sometimes patients who are unfit can be treated in the main theatre where there are better resuscitation facilities.

Contraindications to anaesthesia for ECT
- Old age alone is no reason to refuse treatment.
- Patients with severe hypertension, myocardial ischaemia, stenotic valvular disease or aortic aneurysm have to be considered carefully because of the anaesthetic risk.

- Glaucoma is an absolute contraindication because intra-ocular pressure rises during treatment.
- Thrombophlebitis is contraindicated unless anti-coagulated.
- Raised intracranial pressure is hazardous and, if suspected, fundal inspection should be carried out.
- Treatment should be delayed until 3 months after myocardial infarction.
- Upper airway obstruction is an absolute contra-indication to treatment.
- A patient who has had a cerebrovascular accident within the last 3 months should not have treatment.

Administration of ECT

ECT was first used in 1938, and has remained an effective treatment for depression. Recovery rates of 80 per cent can be expected. Junior doctors find themselves on the ECT rota and can feel quite wary of this procedure, which has received so much attention from the media.

The Royal College of Psychiatrists has drawn up an instruction manual and a video which all clinicians should consult before starting to give the treatment. There is also a consultant who is responsible for ECT, and he or she should be present initially until the junior doctor gains confidence in the procedure. It also helps to have an experienced ECT nurse available who is familiar with the equipment and who ensures that everything is in good working order

Treatment schedule

Two aspects of treatment need to be considered, namely the *frequency* and *total number* of treatments.

In the USA it is common to administer ECT three times weekly, but in the UK twice a week is the usual practice. The average number of treatments also varies. According to the national survey conducted by Pippard and Ellem, 6.5 was the median number of treatments given, and in the USA the average is 9 treatments. There does not appear to be any difference in outcome, and further research suggests that three times weekly may be more useful.

The ECT suite should include a separate waiting area, a treatment area, a recovery area and a further waiting area. It should be pleasant and reasonably spacious. The patient should present fasting and having given consent, as described previously. The procedure is most often received as an in-patient, but occasionally it can be used for outpatients, so long as the patient has someone accompanying him or her. After the anaesthetist has induced anaesthesia, the psychiatrist places the electrodes on the scalp either bitemporally for bilateral treatment, or in the unilateral position.

Once contact has been established (most modern machines will indicate this), the button is pressed and the length of the seizure is recorded.

Cuff method
A cuff is inflated above systolic pressure, on the arm which is not being used by the anaesthetist, and is left inflated throughout the treatment so that the arm is unaffected by the muscle relaxant.

EEG monitoring
This is the most direct method of assessing seizure activity, and it rarely underestimates the seizure length. However, it is not widely used in the UK.

An adequate seizure at the first treatment session should:
• be generalized – however, because of the muscle relaxant you may not observe much other than movement of the eyebrows and up-going plantars;

- start with a tonic phase after a possible latent period;
- be in clonic phase;
- last for 15 s or more peripherally, or 25 s on EEG recording.

Older ECT machines were sine wave, and it was common procedure to have a standard setting for every patient. This resulted in unnecessary cognitive side-effects. Newer machines such as the Ectron 5A and Mecta SRI machines have brief pulse stimuli and the dose can be titrated according to the needs of the patient.

The term 'seizure threshold' refers to the minimum instrument setting required to induce a generalized seizure. This is affected by factors which raise the seizure threshold and tend to shorten the seizure, including age, sex, medication and modality of ECT (unilateral/bilateral).

Medications which decrease seizures include:

- benzodiazepines;
- anticonvulsants;
- anaesthetic drugs.

Medications which increase seizures include:

- alcohol;
- caffeine;
- SSRIs;
- TCAs.

Once the approximate seizure threshold is known, the dose is increased at the next treatment. The dose will probably increase during the course of the treatment by as much as 80 per cent. It may be necessary to re-stimulate if the supra-threshold is not reached initially. The anaesthetist should be warned in this case.

19

TALKING TO RELATIVES — ISSUES OF CONFIDENTIALITY

Families, friends and neighbours play a major role in the care of people with mental health problems. The White Paper entitled *Caring for People* (Department of Health, 1989. London: HMSO) set out to ensure that service providers make practical support for carers a high priority.

Community care often depends on contributions by families and voluntary groups. Therefore it is important that these same families and voluntary groups are involved in the planning of services, and that there is a clear role demarcation between them and professional staff; otherwise, they may feel overwhelmed and professionals may feel that they are taking on too much.

If carers/relatives are to take responsibility for housing the patient, encouraging appropriate behaviour and supervising their medication, as well as reporting signs of relapse, they need to be educated about the illness and they also need to be well supported, with someone to call in an emergency.

It is difficult for the professionals to fulfil their roles with respect to the patient and his or her relatives, as there is often conflict about confidentiality. Confidentiality is particularly important in psychiatry because highly sensitive information is often collected. In general, the psychiatrist should seek the consent of the patient before he or she asks for information from a carer or relative.

Sometimes the patient is too disturbed to give a coherent account of events, and this information is important, so the psychiatrist should use discretion when seeking information from someone else (use close relatives rather than employers or colleagues). Similarly, when relatives or carers need information, consent should be given by the patient prior to the disclosure of such information.

Sometimes the relatives' role can become destructive. They may become too critical or over-protective and not give the patient any privacy or autonomy. Research has shown that this increases the chances of relapse, and high expressed emotion should be discouraged by educating the relative and if necessary encouraging the patient to move out of their care.

It is commonplace for relatives/carers to be involved with discharge plans in the Care Programme Approach, and to be present at meetings.

It is important not to give information out over the telephone to someone who claims to be a close relative without seeking the consent of the patient and arranging for a face-to-face meeting with the relative and if possible the patient.

In the UK, the GMC has issued guidelines on situations in which confidentiality may be breached by doctors. Doctors may give information to the police when the patient is causing concern for public safety or is making threats to an identified person. Threats to kill or harm a relative or partner should be taken seriously, and consideration for their safety is important. In this situation it is reasonable to disclose sufficient information to the person under threat.

20

RELATIONSHIPS WITH OTHER HOSPITAL DEPARTMENTS

Hospital liaison psychiatry relates to the role of psychiatrists in general hospitals with respect to physical disorders occurring in conjunction with psychiatric/psychological disorders. Core activities of a good hospital liaison psychiatry service, in which trainee psychiatrists should therefore ensure that they gain adequate clinical experience and theoretical knowledge, include the following:

1. the psychiatric assessment of patients with physical disorders;
2. the psychiatric assessment and management of patients who have harmed themselves or who have threatened to harm themselves;
3. giving advice to specialized medical services, including those involved with:
   - endocrinology;
   - neurology;
   - neurosurgery;
   - cardiothoracic surgery;
   - nephrology;
   - intensive care;
   - special care baby units;
   - accident and emergency;
   - HIV infection;
   - haematology;
   - radiotherapy and oncology;
4. pain management;
5. complications of psychoactive substance misuse and dependence;

6. hypochondriasis and disorders presenting with symptoms of physical disorders;
7. care of the dying and the bereaved;
8. hospital staff interactions.

An important point to bear in mind is that other hospital departments may entertain unreal expectations of the psychiatrist. It is important, for example, not immediately to offer to take over care of a patient on a medical or surgical ward who is suffering from an acute confusional state; the cause is usually physical, and this should first be discovered and managed by the medical or surgical team. It is useful to hold joint ward rounds with the other departments being covered by your team. As well as aiding communication about patients, joint ward rounds help you to relate better to the staff from other departments. If the doctors from both the psychiatric teams and other departments achieve a situation whereby they are all 'speaking the same language' and they have the same objectives, and if the physicians/surgeons know that the liaison psychiatrists are available, then this in turn should increase the coping skills of the former.

PATIENTS WHO WILL NOT EAT OR DRINK

This problem frequently presents as a difficult issue in liaison psychiatry.

Aetiology

1. The most common cause of failure to eat or drink is untreated depression. The patient may have been admitted to a medical ward following prolonged anorexia and weight loss, or it may be an acute phenomenon following a traumatic period in the patient's life. The majority of people who present in this way are elderly, and many of them do not survive.
2. Patients may refuse food or fluids because of difficulty in swallowing, and they may be afraid of choking. This may be episodic, or may only

occur with food of certain consistencies, and may therefore not be detected.

3. Some people refuse to eat because they are angry about being in hospital or they do not like the food. They often do not appreciate how harmful this behaviour can be to them.

A recent case involved a 70-year-old woman who had accidentally walked in front of a motorcycle. She survived, but with serious injuries. She contracted multiple resistant *Staphylococcus aureus* and *Clostridium welchi*. As a consequence of this she was isolated for 3 months. She became very angry and stopped eating and drinking. She failed to appreciate the damage she was doing to herself, and she would pull out any nasogastric tubes. The gastroenterology department experienced some problem in inserting a percutaneous endoscopic gastrotomy (PEG) tube in a patient with what they perceived to be a treatable depression. The patient was not expected to live, but she showed a dramatic improvement following transfer from her barrier-nursed room to a dormitory ward.

Presentation is with increasing weight loss, with or without dehydration. Often such patients drink fluids for a longer period of time. It is important that a working diagnosis is established and that *food* and *fluids* are given in the mean time either by nasogastric tube or preferably by PEG tube. Most such patients are given antidepressants, and sometimes a very short course of steroids will stimulate the appetite so that they start to eat again.

The prognosis is poor if the situation persists and no one takes responsibility for instituting an adequate calorie and fluid intake.

21

OUT-PATIENT CLINICS

Aspects of the monitoring of patients taking particular medications are considered here.

Lithium

Since lithium is excreted mainly by the kidneys, check the patient's renal function before starting him or her on lithium therapy. This usually entails assessing the plasma urea, electrolytes and creatinine levels. However, if there is any suggestion of poor renal function, full renal function studies must be carried out.

Regular monitoring of plasma lithium levels is required once a patient is started on lithium therapy because lithium has a low therapeutic index. Plasma levels are estimated 8 to 12 hours after the preceding dose, and the dose is adjusted to achieve a lithium level of between 0.4 and 1.0 mmol L^{-1} for prophylactic purposes. The lower levels are required in the elderly. Plasma lithium concentrations are checked up to twice weekly when lithium therapy is first started. In established maintenance lithium therapy the frequency of plasma monitoring can be reduced to once every 3 months. Plasma urea, electrolytes and creatinine levels should be checked at the same time in order to monitor renal function. Thyroid function tests should be checked every 6 months (thyroid function disturbances can result from long-term lithium therapy).

Antipsychotics

Practical aspects of treating out-patients with clozapine or with antipsychotic depot preparations are considered in Chapter 17 (Psychotropic Medication).

Carbamazepine

According to the British National Formulary (BNF), the monitoring of plasma concentrations may be helpful in determining optimum dosage.

Cyproterone acetate

Check the patient's blood count and liver function tests prior to starting treatment with this drug. During treatment the blood count and liver function tests should be monitored regularly.

Discharge

22

DISCHARGE PLANNING AND
COMMUNITY CARE

Since the early 1970s patients have been moving into the community from mental hospitals and the difficulties have increased with regard to treatment of people with serious mental illness who are not available and under observation 24 hours a day.

A document was issued by the Department of Health requiring mental health providers to formulate a policy in relation to the care programme approach (CPA) by April 1991. The care programme approach is a formalized discharge plan for patients suffering from serious mental illness, and it aims to ensure that they receive a co-ordinated package of care in the community.

A CPA is the result of a needs-based multiprofessional assessment which is health led and ensures that a key worker is allocated to each patient. Care management, the Social Services arm of the co-ordinated care packages, should if possible be merged.

There are various levels of CPA. One level applies to patients who are found to have limited disability and whose support needs are therefore low and likely to remain stable. They may only be in contact with one practitioner, who will be the CPA key worker.

Other patients require a more complex care package and are involved with several members of one or more teams. Indications for this level of CPA are:

- individuals who have suffered from serious mental illness in the past or who continue to suffer from it;
- individuals who are mentally ill and who are thought to have a poor prognosis;
- patients discharged according to the terms of Section 117 of the Mental Health Act (MHA) 1983 (who have been admitted under Section 3 MHA 1983);
- patients who have been discharged following an admission of longer than 3 months;
- patients who have had three or more separate admissions in the previous 18 months;
- patients with a diagnosis of dementia, who are discharged to their own homes and are thought to be at risk;
- patients who have made a serious suicide attempt and have concomitant mental illness;
- patients who are 'difficult' or who are offenders.

Supervision Register – Section 25 MHA 1983
The decision as to whether a patient should be placed on the supervision register rests with the RMO or consultant responsible for the patient's care. This decision should be made in consultation with the other members of the multidisciplinary team who are involved in the patient's care.

Patients should be included if it is felt that:
- they have a serious mental illness;
- they are likely to be at significant risk of commiting serious violence;
- they are likely to be at significant risk of suicide or self-neglect.

Risk assessment should be of the type described in *Guidance on the discharge of mentally disordered people and continuing care in the community* (HSG (94) 27). Risk assessment should consider (i) the past history of the patient, (ii) self-reporting by the patient at interview and (iii) observation of the patient's behaviour and mental state. Discrepancies between what the patient says and what is observed should be noted. Statistics derived from studies of related cases should also be considered, as they may be prediction indicators.

23

LETTERS TO GENERAL PRACTITIONERS AND OTHER PROFESSIONALS

▬

General practitioners

In general the discharge letter that is sent to a patient's general practitioner should be kept short. It should outline the main points regarding the patient's:

- diagnosis;
- management;
- future management.

There are several advantages in not sending long, detailed psychiatric case reports to general practitioners:

- most general practitioners are very busy;
- general practitioners are usually already familiar with most of the background information about their patients;
- a short discharge letter can more easily be filed with the general practitioner's other notes on their patient.

Other professionals

Letters to other professionals should reflect the amount of detail that they require, within the bounds of patient confidentiality. Thus a referral letter to a dermatologist may be relatively short and would not usually need to refer to the patient's educational history, while a referral letter to a social worker should describe in detail the social aspects

of the patient. Similarly, while a letter to a local
council confirming the need for housing for a
patient would not normally need to refer to the
patient's psychosexual history or any other confidential non-relevant material, this is clearly not
the case for a letter of referral to a psycho-
therapist.

Part
IV

Common Medical and Psychiatric Emergencies and Procedures

24

EMERGENCIES

SUICIDAL RISK

SUICIDAL IDEAS OR THOUGHTS

Assessment

Patients should be asked about any suicidal thoughts or ideas they have. Doing this does not cause the idea of suicide to enter the patient's mind for the first time. Questions asked can progressively home in on any suicidal thoughts, starting with a general open-ended question asking how the patient sees the future, through more specific questions such as 'Have you ever thought life was not worth living?', and finally, if appropriate, questions about any specific suicidal plans the patient may have. Any evidence from the patient that he or she feels there is no future, that life is pointless, or that suicide is being considered should be taken extremely seriously.

Look for evidence of any of the following psychiatric and physical illnesses that are associated with an increased risk of suicide:

- depressive episodes – bear in mind that depressed patients may use their antidepressants to try to kill themselves – this is particularly worrying in the case of tricyclic antidepressants and MAOIs;
- alcohol dependence;
- other psychoactive substance use disorders, particularly illicit drug use;
- personality disorder;
- chronic neuroses;

- schizophrenia, particularly in young men with low mood;
- chronic painful illnesses;
- epilepsy.

Interview the patient and his or her relatives and friends and obtain information about any losses that might increase the risk of suicide, including:

- breakup of a relationship;
- death of a relative or close friend;
- job loss;
- financial loss;
- loss of position or status in society, e.g. because of being arrested for shoplifting.

Also look for evidence of loneliness and reduced or no social contacts.

Management

Important points in the management of a patient with a serious risk of suicide include the following:

- the patient should almost always be admitted as an in-patient – this may have to be a compulsory admission;
- establish a good rapport with the patient, and between the patient and the nursing staff;
- encourage the patient to articulate his or her feelings and thoughts;
- remove any objects that could be used in a suicide attempt, e.g. belts, sharp objects;
- tailor the frequency of observation to the level of risk, and write this in the case-notes as well as informing the nursing staff – e.g. continuous observation if the patient is at high risk;
- nurse the patient in their night-clothes during the day – do not allow the patient to have a pyjama cord or shoe-laces;
- treat any underlying psychiatric or physical disorder;
- bear in mind that patients with psychomotor retardation may be at greater risk as their symptoms improve (e.g. during a course of ECT), as

they may then have the energy to go through with their suicide plans.

FOLLOWING PARASUICIDE/DELIBERATE SELF-HARM

Assessment

During the interview with the patient following an act of parasuicide, ascertain the degree of suicidal intent. A high level of intent is indicated by the following:

1. the act was planned and preparations were made for it;
2. precautions were taken to avoid discovery, and the act was carried out in isolation;
3. the patient did not seek help after the act;
4. the act involved a dangerous method such as:
   - hanging;
   - electrocution;
   - shooting;
   - jumping from a height;
   - drowning;
5. there was a final act such as making a will or leaving a suicide note before the attempt.

Ask the patient to describe their reaction when they discovered that they were not going to die; a high suicide risk is indicated when the patient regrets not having died and still wishes to do so.

Other details that should be obtained in the assessment include:

- the presence of a psychiatric disorder associated with suicide risk;
- a previous history of suicide attempts;
- the patient's current problems;
- the patient's social and financial support upon which he or she can rely.

Management

Treat the patient medically, as appropriate, and carry out a full assessment. Treat any psychiatric disorder.

Factors associated with a repeated attempt of parasuicide/deliberate self-harm include:

- a previous act of parasuicide/deliberate self-harm;
- previous psychiatric treatment;
- dyssocial or antisocial personality disorder;
- alcohol dependence;
- other psychoactive substance use disorder;
- criminal record;
- low social class;
- unemployment.

Following an act of parasuicide/deliberate self-harm, there is a markedly increased risk of committing suicide in the following year, of approximately 100 times that in the general population. Factors associated with an increased risk of suicide following parasuicide/deliberate self-harm include:

1. high suicidal intent – this is elicited in the assessment (see above);
2. psychiatric disorder, in particular;
   - depressive episodes;
   - alcohol dependence;
   - other psychoactive substance use disorders;
   - schizophrenia;
   - dyssocial or antisocial personality disorder;
3. history of previous suicide attempt(s);
4. living in social isolation;
5. age over 45 years;
6. male sex;
7. being unemployed or retired;
8. chronic painful illness.

If the patient is at high risk of suicide then management should be as indicated in the previous subsection.

PEOPLE AT RISK OF SUICIDE

Junior doctors will quite often be called upon to assess the risk of suicide because:

1. those who go on to complete suicide often tell people, including health professionals, that they are planning suicide;
2. it is thought that people remain ambivalent about killing themselves until the end.

Thus it is worth working out your own attitude to suicide prevention and being familiar with procedures employed locally in looking after those at risk.

Suicide prevention is both possible and worthwhile. Sometimes people may feel that suicide is appropriate because a judgement is made that an individual's life is not worth continuing. This view can rarely be justified, and is often perceived by the suicidal person as the final rejection.

It is important not to become angry or abusive when confronted by a patient who appears to be weak willed and/or attention seeking. With appropriate help and care such a patient can become hopeful again and no longer be suicidal.

Suicide prevention in hospital

Important factors include:
- environment – adequate basic facilities; note that bank holidays and other interruptions of daily routine represent an extra hazard;
- nursing staff – levels and training, including resuscitation;
- morale of staff – good morale tends to lead to better communication;
- attitude of staff – good education can challenge negative attitudes.

Levels of observation
The following should be observed:
- appearance;
- general behaviour;
- expression of suicidal ideas, hopelessness, other morbid ideations;
- mood and attitude;
- orientation, memory function;

- insight into present situation; beware of improvement where life crises are unresolved.

Decisions need to be taken about the severity of the risk and which level of observation is needed:

- level 1 – constant, within arm's length;
- level 2 – 15-minute observation (experience has shown that the observations should not take place at regular, and therefore predictable, intervals);
- level 3 – someone (a designated nurse) always knowing the whereabouts of the patient.

RISK OF HARM TO OTHER PEOPLE

ASSESSMENT

Guidelines produced by the Royal College of Psychiatrists (*Assessment and Clinical Management of Risk of Harm to Other People*, Council Report CR53, published in 1996) recommend that, in assessing the risk of harm being caused to other people by a psychiatric patient, the standard psychiatric assessment should include the following.

History
The following areas should be covered:
- previous violence and/or suicidal behaviour;
- evidence of rootlessness or 'social restlessness', e.g. few relationships, frequent changes of address or employment;
- evidence of poor compliance with treatment or disengagement from psychiatric aftercare;
- presence of substance misuse or other potential disinhibiting factors, e.g. a social background promoting violence;
- identification of any precipitants and any changes in mental state or behaviour that have occurred prior to violence and/or relapse.

It should be ascertained whether the following risk factors are stable, or if any have changed recently:

- evidence of recent severe stress, particularly of loss events or the threat of loss;
- evidence of recent discontinuation of medication.

Environment
- Does the patient have access to potential victims, particularly individuals identified in mental state abnormalities?

Mental State Examination
The following should be considered:
- evidence of any threat/control override symptoms: firmly held beliefs of persecution by others (persecutory delusions), or of the mind or body being controlled or interfered with by external forces (delusions of passivity);
- emotions related to violence, e.g. irritability, anger, hostility, suspiciousness;
- specific threats made by the patient.

Conclusion
A formulation should be made based on these and all other items of the history and Mental State Examination, and it should specify both factors that are likely to increase the risk of dangerous behaviour and those which are likely to decrease it. It should aim to answer the following questions.
1. Have I all the information needed, and do I know what the risks are?
2. Are these risks necessary?
3. Have I got enough time to make the right decision?
4. What do I hope will be realized by my actions?

MANAGEMENT OF RISK

The Royal College of Psychiatrists (*Assessment and Clinical Management of Risk of Harm to Other People*, Council Report CR53, 1996) recommends that the clinical management of risk should include the following.

General principles

There are two main principles:

- a clinician, having identified the risk of dangerous behaviour, has a responsibility to take action with a view to ensuring that risk is reduced and managed effectively;
- the management plan should change the balance between risk and safety, following the principles of negotiating safety.

Management plan

Consider where the patient should be managed.

- Is admission as an in-patient necessary?
- Should the patient be detained in hospital?
- What level of physical security is necessary?
- What level of observation is required?
- How should medication be used?
- How should (further) episodes of violence be managed?

If care other than as an in-patient is being considered, the following questions should be asked.

- Has the Care Programme Approach (in the UK) been implemented?
- Has the use of legal powers (mental health legislation, e.g. the Mental Health Act in England and Wales) been considered?
- Is inclusion on the supervision register appropriate?
- What community supports are available, e.g. family, carers, community mental health nurses, social workers, probation service?
- Do the carers and family have access to appropriate support and help?
- Have the carers (professional and lay) and family been adequately informed about the services needed and how they can be accessed? Are they realistic in their expectations?

DEALING WITH VERBAL ABUSE

Although there have been many studies of violent behaviour it is very difficult to find articles dealing with verbal abuse, which can be a prodromal symptom of violence.

Verbal abuse can be defined as speech directed towards a person or persons in a way that warns, intimidates or constitutes an attack on those to whom it is directed.

Psychiatry might be expected to encounter more of this type of behaviour, but in reality all aspects of the medical profession (and other professions) receive their fair share. It is a neglected topic because of the stigma attached to its expression.

Verbal abuse can be received from:
• patients;
• relatives;
• professionals outside one's organization;
• colleagues;
• government.

Verbal abuse from psychiatric patients may have multiple aetiologies which can include:
• irritability – associated with depression, fear, anxiety or alcohol abuse;
• personality disorders such as borderline personality disorder, antisocial personality disorder, histrionic and narcissistic disorder often result in severe forms of verbal abuse;
• paranoia and schizophrenia;
• epilepsy – prodromal irritability linked with suspiciousness and sensitivity, often resulting in verbal abuse, is a recognized symptom of temporal lobe epilepsy;
• Gilles de la Tourette's syndrome is an organic disorder in which the patient experiences a spasmodic tic and may simultaneously swear;
• 'hostility' has been described as a prolonged phase in the recovery from major depressive

illness, and this often leads to verbal abuse. Clinical practice has no place for verbal abuse and does not often figure in the Mental State Examination, although it has strong links with mood disturbance.

Coping with verbal abuse is often easier when it comes from a patient who can readily be understood as 'ill', although it is important not to over-medicalize unpleasant behaviour so that it is no longer attributable to free will. It is closely associated with intellectual and cognitive factors such as value judgements, self-esteem and expectations. The Patient's Charter and frequent encouragement in the press to complain about the health service when it is less than perfect may encourage some people to feel that the normal social constraints do not apply to them.

Colleagues may have different expectations from a professional, which are not included in that professional's job description.

It is important when subjected to verbal abuse not to 'bite the one who bites', as counselled by Seneca, but it also reasonable not to take this for granted as part of the job. Retaliation is unhelpful and a calm reasonable tone of voice, if it can be achieved, should be adopted. A recognition of why verbal abuse is happening at this particular moment in time can sometimes be achieved by studying the dynamics of the situation.

However, in order to avoid escalating stress in the workplace, adequate support and understanding must be present. If no support is forthcoming, it is advisable to adopt measures to decrease stress, such as talking about the abuse to your tutor or a friend. Adequate time away from the working environment is important, as it is easy to get things out of perspective after a busy weekend on call.

THE VIOLENT PATIENT

Precautions

Precautions that can be taken to reduce the risk of physical violence by a patient towards you include the following:

- ensure that other members of staff always know whom you will be interviewing and where the interview will take place;
- make sure that you are familiar with your ward/hospital policies on violence;
- make sure that you are familiar with the location of alarm buttons and alarm bells;
- it is useful to obtain training in simple breakaway techniques at an early stage in your first psychiatric placement;
- remove any potential weapons (e.g. letter-openers) from the interview area;
- sit about 1 metre from the patient, at the same level as him or her, and in a position in which you can always look at the patient but the patient can look away, i.e. sit at right angles to each other;
- sit nearer the door, so that it is less likely that the patient could trap you in the room; however, the patient should also have free access to the door, so that he or she does not feel trapped.

The threatening patient

If a patient does become acutely angry or threatening, the following points can be helpful in reducing the risk of physical violence by him or her:

- adopt a calm manner;
- talk in a quiet voice – do not shout back;
- avoid direct eye contact;
- keep at the same level or even lower than the patient – sit rather than stand so that he or she does not feel overwhelmed;
- do not talk down to the patient, and take into account any delusion(s) from which he or she is suffering, e.g. sometimes smiling can be difficult

as the patient may believe he or she is being laughed at;

- terminate the interview as soon as you reasonably can, but be prepared to talk with the patient for a prolonged period before he or she becomes more relaxed.

OTHER EMERGENCIES

DELIRIUM

Delirium is characterized by acute generalized psychological dysfunction that usually fluctuates in degree. Impairment of consciousness occurs, often accompanied by abnormal perceptions and mood changes.

Clinical features

Prodromal symptoms
These may include:

- being perplexed and agitated;
- hypersensitivity to light;
- hypersensitivity to sound.

Delirium
The main symptoms are as follows:

- being perplexed, anxious, agitated or depressed;
- acute onset;
- fluctuating level of consciousness – often worse at night;
- illusions;
- hallucinations (visual, auditory and/or tactile);
- delusions – these may be persecutory;
- poor concentration;
- disorientation in time and place;
- impairment of memory (including impairment of new learning, registration, retention and recall).

Management

Investigations

Carry out appropriate investigations to determine the underlying cause, which should be treated.

Nursing

1. Good, calming nursing care is required, preferably in a quiet single room.
2. Explain the nature of the condition to the patient; this should help to:
   • reassure the patient;
   • reduce the effects of illusions, hallucinations and delusions.
3. Reduce the effects of disorientation, e.g. by:
   • allowing the patient to know the time;
   • placing a television in the room;
   • allowing visitors.
4. Use a low level of lighting at night, which:
   • reassures the patient of their orientation in place;
   • does not interfere with sleep.

Fluid and electrolyte balance

Ensure that the patient has an adequate fluid and electrolyte balance.

Medication

• In patients without hepatic failure, oral or intramuscular haloperidol may be used if the patient is very agitated, anxious or frightened.
• In patients with hepatic failure, benzodiazepines may be used instead of haloperidol.
• Benzodiazepines may be given as a hypnotic at night.

OCULOGYRIC CRISIS

Clinical features

This is an acute, often painful, involuntary spasm of the extra-ocular muscles, often causing movement of the eyes superiorly and to one side. It is an acute dystonic reaction, usually occurring soon after commencing pharmacotherapy with antipsychotic medication.

Management

The immediate treatment of a drug-induced oculogyric crisis is the same as that of any other antipsychotic-induced acute dystonic reaction, namely the administration parenterally of an antimuscarinic drug, such as:

- 5–10 mg procyclidine by intramuscular injection, repeated if necessary after 20 minutes (maximum 20 mg/day), *or*;
- 5 mg procyclidine by intravenous injection, which is usually effective within 5 minutes, *or*;
- 1–2 mg benztropine by intramuscular or intravenous injection.

After the immediate management, consider reducing the antipsychotic dose or changing the type of antipsychotic.

NEUROLEPTIC MALIGNANT SYNDROME

Clinical features

Neuroleptic malignant syndrome is characterized by:

1. hyperthermia;
2. fluctuating level of consciousness;
3. muscular rigidity;
4. autonomic dysfunction:
   - tachycardia;
   - labile blood pressure;
   - pallor;
   - sweating;
   - urinary incontinence.

Investigations

Laboratory investigations in neuroleptic malignant syndrome commonly, but not invariably, demonstrate:

- elevated creatinine phosphokinase;

- elevated white blood count;
- abnormal liver function tests.

Management

Neuroleptic malignant syndrome is potentially fatal and requires urgent medical treatment. The patient should be referred to the physicians and transferred to a medical ward, where the management should include the following:

1. withdraw psychotropic medication, particularly antipsychotics, antidepressants and lithium (even with treatment, the syndrome may be prolonged if a depot antipsychotic preparation has been administered);
2. check:
   - white blood count;
   - urea and electrolytes;
   - creatinine phosphokinase;
   - liver function tests;
3. rehydration;
4. correction of pyrexia;
5. consider treatment with bromocriptine (a dopamine agonist) and dantrolene (a muscle relaxant);
6. benzodiazepines are not contraindicated for sedation.

EMERGENCY CONTRACEPTION

Following unprotected sexual intercourse, care should be taken to exclude any sexually transmitted diseases.

Hormonal method

Method

Within 72 hours (3 days) of unprotected sexual intercourse, 2 tablets are taken each containing 50 μg ethinyloestradiol and 250 μg levonorgestrel. Exactly 12 hours later a further 2 tablets are taken each containing 50 μg ethinyloestradiol and 250 μg levonorgestrel. (In the UK, these tablets for post-coital contraception are available in a 4-tablet pack as Schering PC4®, from Schering Health.)

If the patient vomits within 3 hours of taking the 2 tablets, consider either giving 2 replacement tablets with an anti-emetic (not metoclopramide) or using the IUD method (see below).

The patient should be seen urgently if she develops lower abdominal pain or heavy bleeding.

Contraindications
These include:
• history of thrombosis;
• focal migraine at the time of presentation.

Side-effects
These include:
• nausea and vomiting;
• headache;
• dizziness;
• breast discomfort;
• menstrual irregularities.

IUD method
Method
This method is more effective than the above hormonal method, and involves the insertion of an intrauterine contraceptive device within 120 hours (5 days) of unprotected sexual intercourse. If more than 5 days have passed, the IUD can still be inserted up to 5 days following the earliest likely calculated date of ovulation.

Contraindications
These include:
1. severe anaemia;
2. immunosuppressive therapy;
3. in the case of copper IUDs:
   • copper allergy;
   • Wilson's disease;

- medical diathermy.

Side-effects

These include:

- uterine perforation;
- cervical perforation;
- exacerbation of pelvic infection;
- hypersensitivity;
- pain – on insertion;
- bleeding – on insertion;
- epileptic seizure – on insertion;
- vasovagal attack – on insertion.

PREGNANCY TESTS

Early pregnancy and pregnancy failure (e.g. ectopic pregnancy) can be tested for using high-resolution ultrasound scanning and/or biochemical diagnosis. The latter usually involves the assay of beta human chorionic gonadotrophin (βhCG) which can be detected in maternal blood 7–9 days following conception, and in urine 1 to 2 days later.

POISONING

Management

Admission

Any patient suspected of having taken an overdose or being otherwise poisoned should be admitted immediately to a general hospital (accident & emergency or general medicine). Their care should be carried out by doctors with the appropriate experience. If in doubt, never hesitate to ask for expert advice (e.g. from a physician or the Poisons Information Centre).

Type of poison

The nature of the poison and probable amount both need to be identified. TICTAC, a computerized tablet and capsule identification system, may be used in the UK and Eire via a Regional Drug Information Centre or Poisons Information Centre (see below).

General medical care

Specific information is available in the UK and Eire from a Poisons Information Centre. The BNF is also a very useful source of information.

Specific drugs

Paracetamol

Urgent medical admission is required following a suspected paracetamol overdose. Even if there are few symptoms initially, the patient may develop potentially fatal hepatocellular necrosis within 4 days. The following initial blood tests should be carried out, usually by physicians or accident & emergency staff:

- urea and electrolytes;
- paracetamol;
- liver function tests;
- glucose;
- clotting screen.

Gastric lavage is worth attempting within 2 hours of ingestion. Within 12 hours of ingestion, antidotes (e.g. acetylcysteine, methionine) may protect the liver.

Aspirin

Urgent medical admission is required following a suspected aspirin overdose. Note that the absorption may be delayed in the case of enteric-coated tablets. Important clinical features of salicylate poisoning include:

- hyperventilation;
- tinnitus;
- deafness;
- vasodilatation;
- sweating;
- coma – in the case of severe poisoning.

The following initial blood tests should be carried out, usually by physicians or accident and emergency staff:

- urea and electrolytes;
- salicylate;
- acid-base state;
- clotting screen.

Gastric lavage is worth attempting within 4 hours of ingestion. Other measures, as appropriate, may include the use of activated charcoal, forced alkaline diuresis (although not if the patient has poor renal or cardiac function), and haemodialysis.

Opioids

Urgent medical admission is required following a suspected opioid overdose. Important clinical features of opioid poisoning include:

- pinpoint pupils;
- coma;
- respiratory depression.

It is important to assess:

- pulse;
- blood pressure;
- respiratory rate and depth;
- pupil size.

Management includes the use of the antidote naloxone.

Tricyclic antidepressants

Medical admission is strongly advised following a suspected tricyclic antidepressant overdose. Important dangerous consequences of tricyclic antidepressant poisoning include:

- cardiac conduction defects;
- cardiac arrhythmias.

Other clinical features may include:

- dry mouth;
- coma;
- hypotension;
- hyperthermia;

- hyperreflexia;
- extensor plantar responses;
- convulsions;
- respiratory failure;
- mydriasis;
- urinary retention.

The following initial blood tests should be carried out, usually by physicians or accident & emergency staff:

- urea and electrolytes;
- blood gases;
- acid-base state.

Management includes activated charcoal by mouth, supportive measures to ensure a patent airway and adequate ventilation during transfer to a medical ward, cardiac monitoring, intravenous diazepam if the patient convulses, and correction of hypoxia and acidosis. (Anti-arrhythmic drugs should be avoided.)

Benzodiazepines

A benzodiazepine overdose is not usually life-threatening. However, expert advice should be sought if there are any complicating factors or any other cause for concern. Clinical features of benzodiazepine poisoning include:

- drowsiness;
- ataxia;
- dysarthria;
- impaired consciousness.

If respiratory depression is suspected, then arterial blood gases should be monitored.

Lithium

The features of lithium toxicity are listed in Chapter 17 (Psychotropic Medication). Its management includes diuresis, monitoring fluid and electrolyte balance, monitoring renal function, and controlling convulsions. Severe toxicity may require haemodialysis.

Phenothiazines

Clinical features of phenothiazine poisoning include:

- impaired consciousness;
- respiratory depression;
- hypotension;
- hypothermia;
- sinus tachycardia;
- cardiac arrhythmias;
- convulsions.

Management includes monitoring respiration and blood pressure, maintaining the airway, and cardiac monitoring. Cardiac arrhythmias may require pharmacotherapy if they do not respond to the correction of hypoxia and acidosis.

Poisons information centres

In the UK, information is available 24 hours a day on poisoning from the following poisons information centres:

Belfast	Tel: (01232) 240503
Birmingham	Tel: (0121) 5075588
	Tel: (0121) 5075589
Cardiff	Tel: (01222) 709901
Dublin	Tel: Dublin 8379964
	Tel: Dublin 8379966
Edinburgh	Tel: (0131) 5362300
Leeds	Tel: (0113) 2430715
	Tel: (0113) 2923547
London	Tel: (0171) 6359191
	Tel: (0171) 9555095
Newcastle upon Tyne	Tel: (0191) 2325131

RESUSCITATION

Ensure that you know the cardiac arrest emergency number for your hospital, and also that you know how to give details of your location in the hospital.

You should attend a life support training course regularly (at least annually). Ensure that you know the location of the resuscitation trolleys and how to use them – it is important to be familiar with the cardiac defibrillator on these trolleys.

Basic life support

Figure 24.1 is a flow chart summarizing the various steps involved in carrying out basic life support in cardiopulmonary resuscitation.

Open the airway:

- undo the patient's tie and any other clothing around the neck;
- open the mouth;
- remove obstructions from the mouth.

Clear the tongue away from the throat by tilting the head and lifting the chin, as shown in Fig. 24.2.

If the patient is unresponsive but is breathing and has a detectable carotid pulse, place him or her

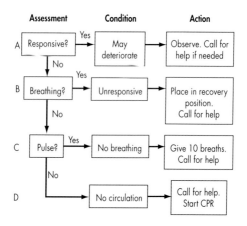

FIGURE 24.1   Summary of basic life support, after the *Guidelines for Basic Life Support* issued by the Basic Life Support Working Party of the European Resuscitation Council.

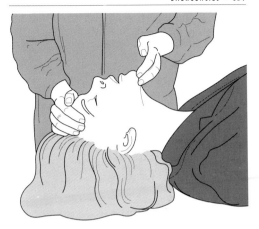

FIGURE 24.2   Head tilt and chin lift (reproduced with permission from Toghill, P.J. (ed.) 1997: *Essential medical procedures*. London: Arnold).

in the recovery position. This is shown in more detail in Fig. 24.3.

If the patient is unresponsive, not breathing spontaneously, and has no detectable carotid pulse, commence cardiopulmonary resuscitation. This is shown in more detail in Fig. 24.4.

Starting with two expired air ventilations, a ratio of air ventilation to chest compression of 2:15 is

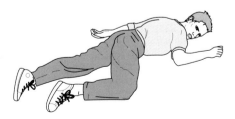

FIGURE 24.3   Recovery position (reproduced with permission from Toghill, P.J. (ed.) 1997: *Essential medical procedures*. London: Arnold).

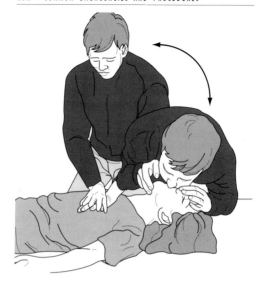

FIGURE 24.4 Chest compression and expired air respiration (reproduced with permission from Toghill, P.J. (ed.) 1997: *Essential medical procedures.* London: Arnold).

carried out. If a second helper is available, they should attempt to summon help.

Advanced life support

Arrhythmias in cardiac arrest

It is important to obtain an ECG recording. You should therefore be familiar with the ECG machine(s) on your resuscitation trolleys, and the positions of the ECG chest electrodes, shown in Fig. 24.5.

In cardiac arrest, the following types of arrhythmia, the typical ECG traces of which are shown in Fig. 24.6, may occur:

• ventricular fibrillation (Fig. 24.6a);
• pulseless ventricular tachycardia (Fig. 24.6b);
• asystole (Fig. 24.6c);

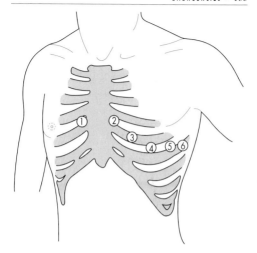

FIGURE 24.5 Position of ECG chest electrodes.

- electromechanical dissociation (Fig. 24.6d).

Ventricular fibrillation or pulseless ventricular tachycardia

The algorithm shown in Fig. 24.7 should be followed in the case of ventricular fibrillation or pulseless ventricular tachycardia.

The following precautions need to be taken before delivering a DC shock using a defibrillator:

- any glyceryl trinitrate patches should be removed in order to avoid burns;
- the electrode jelly or gel pads under each defibrillator paddle should not be in contact with each other in order to avoid short-circuiting;
- if using gel pads, ensure that you know whether these need to be replaced after each DC shock;
- the paddles should not be applied near artificial pacemakers;
- nobody should be in contact with the patient or the bed when the DC shock is to be delivered – if

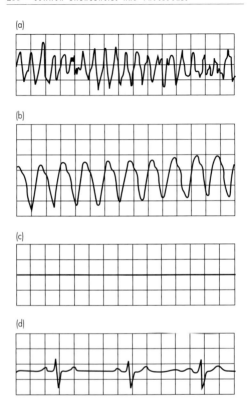

FIGURE 24.6 The ECG appearances of (a) ventricular fibrillation, (b) ventricular tachycardia, (c) asystole and (d) electromechanical dissociation.

FIGURE 24.7 Management algorithm for ventricular fibrillation (VF) or pulseless ventricular tachycardia (VT) (reprinted from *Resuscitation* **24**, Advanced Life Support Working Party of the European Resuscitation Council, Guidelines for advanced life support, 115 (1992), with kind permission from Elsevier Science Ltd, The Boulevard, Langford Lane, Kidlington OX5 1GB, UK).

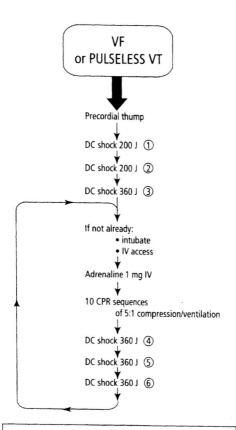

VF
or PULSELESS VT

Precordial thump

DC shock 200 J ①

DC shock 200 J ②

DC shock 360 J ③

If not already:
- intubate
- IV access

Adrenaline 1 mg IV

10 CPR sequences
of 5:1 compression/ventilation

DC shock 360 J ④

DC shock 360 J ⑤

DC shock 360 J ⑥

The interval between shocks 3 and 4 should not be >2 min.
Adrenaline given during loop approx. every 2–3 min.
Continue loops for as long as defibrillation is indicated.
After three loops consider:
- an alkalizing agent,
- an antiarrhythmic agent.

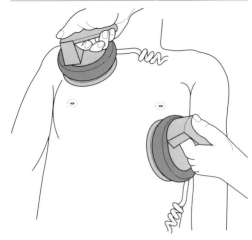

FIGURE 24.8   Standard positions of manual defibrillator paddles (reproduced with permission from Toghill, P.J. (ed.) 1997: *Essential medical procedures*. London: Arnold).

you are delivering the DC shock, ensure that everybody, including you, is standing well clear.

Figure 24.8 shows the standard manual defibrillator paddle positions.

If an intravenous line cannot be established, consider giving double or triple doses of adrenaline via an endotracheal tube.

Asystole
The algorithm shown in Fig. 24.9 should be followed in the case of asystole.

If an intravenous line cannot be established, consider giving double or triple doses of adrenaline or atropine via an endotracheal tube.

FIGURE 24.9   Management algorithm for asystole (reprinted from *Resuscitation* **24**, Advanced Life Support Working Party of the European Resuscitation Council, Guidelines for advanced life support, 118 (1992), with kind permission from Elsevier Science Ltd, The Boulevard, Langford Lane, Kidlington OX5 1GB, UK).

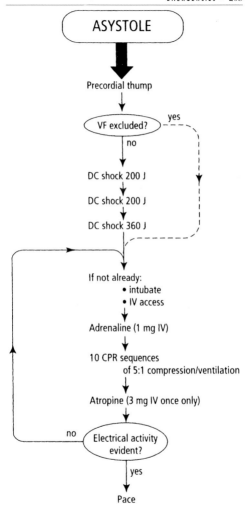

ASYSTOLE

Precordial thump

VF excluded? — yes

no

DC shock 200 J

DC shock 200 J

DC shock 360 J

If not already:
• intubate
• IV access

Adrenaline (1 mg IV)

10 CPR sequences
of 5:1 compression/ventilation

Atropine (3 mg IV once only)

no — Electrical activity
evident?

yes

Pace

Note: If no response after three cycles consider
high-dose adrenaline: 5 mg IV.

Electromechanical dissociation

In electromechanical dissociation there is ECG evidence of electrical activity (QRS complexes) but no

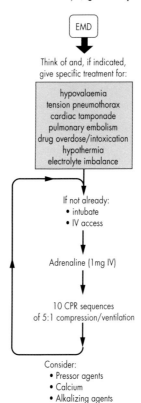

FIGURE 24.10 Management algorithm for electromechanical dissociation (EMD) (reprinted from *Resuscitation* **24**, Advanced Life Support Working Party of the European Resuscitation Council, Guidelines for advanced life support, 120 (1992), with kind permission from Elsevier Science Ltd, The Boulevard, Langford Lane, Kidlington OX5 1GB, UK).

palpable pulse. The algorithm shown in Fig. 24.10 should be followed.

As indicated in Fig. 24.10, you should think of the possible causes of electromechanical dissociation, and give specific treatment for each cause, as follows:

- hypovolaemia – fluid replacement;
- tension pneumothorax – chest drain;
- cardiac tamponade – pericardiocentesis;
- pulmonary embolism – anticoagulant therapy, and consider thrombolysis or pulmonary embolectomy;
- drug overdose/intoxication – see the appropriate subsection in this book;
- hypothermia – warm the patient;
- electrolyte imbalance – monitor and correct imbalance.

If an intravenous line cannot be established, consider giving double or triple doses of adrenaline via an endotracheal tube.

WERNICKE'S ENCEPHALOPATHY

Clinical features

The most important clinical features of Wernicke's encephalopathy are:

- ophthalmoplegia;
- nystagmus;
- ataxia;
- clouding of consciousness;
- peripheral neuropathy.

Management

This includes:

- bed rest – the possibility exists of sudden cardiovascular collapse;
- absention from alcohol;
- treatment with thiamine (vitamin B_1) – note that parenteral administration of B vitamins may be associated with anaphylaxis;

- restrict carbohydrate intake initially – in the presence of vitamin B$_1$ deficiency a carbohydrate intake may worsen this vitamin deficiency, and may itself precipitate Wernicke's encephalopathy.

So far as the parenteral administration of vitamin B$_1$ is concerned, the Committee on Safety of Medicines (CSM) has issued the following advice:

Since potentially serious allergic adverse reactions may occur during or shortly after administration, the CSM has recommended that:

1. use be restricted to patients in whom parenteral treatment is essential;
2. intravenous injections should be administered slowly (over 10 minutes);
3. facilities for treating anaphylaxis should be available when administered.

ACUTE SEVERE ASTHMA

Acute severe asthma in adults

The clinical features of acute severe asthma in adults include:

- persistent dyspnoea – the patient cannot complete sentences;
- pulse $\geq$ 110 beats/minute;
- respiratory rate $\geq$ 25 breaths/minute;
- peak flow $\leq$ 50 per cent of predicted or best.

If two or more of these features are present, the patient should be transferred to the care of the physicians as an in-patient, where initial treatment would typically consist of:

- oxygen 40–60 per cent;
- nebulized salbutamol or nebulized terbutaline;
- oral prednisolone (30–60 mg) or intravenous hydrocortisone (200 mg).

Life-threatening asthma in adults

The clinical features of life-threatening asthma in adults include:

- silent chest;
- cyanosis;
- bradycardia or exhaustion;

• peak flow < 33 per cent of predicted or best.

The patient should immediately be transferred to accident and emergency or a general hospital ward. (Note that the patient may not have all these signs, and indeed may not appear distressed, but the presence of any of these signs should be taken extremely seriously.) Initial treatment includes:

- oral prednisolone (30–60 mg) or intravenous hydrocortisone (200 mg) immediately;
- oxygen-driven nebulizer in the ambulance;
- nebulized β_2 stimulant with nebulized ipratropium *or* subcutaneous terbutaline *or* slow intravenous aminophylline (250 mg) (but do *not* give intravenous aminophylline if the patient is already taking oral theophylline).

If a nebulizer is not available, administer two puffs of β_2 stimulant using a large-volume spacer; repeat 10 to 20 times.

DIABETIC KETOACIDOSIS

Clinical features

The main clinical features of diabetic ketoacidosis are:

1. history of:
   - insufficient insulin intake;
   - infection (particularly renal, respiratory or gastrointestinal);
   - digestive abnormality;
2. slow onset – ill-health for hours or days;
3. confusion;
4. abdominal pain and vomiting;
5. dehydration – dry skin and dry tongue;
6. hypotension and weak pulse;
7. overbreathing;
8. ketones may be smelt in the breath;
9. may progress to coma.

Blood

The main features are:
- hyperglycaemia;

- decreased plasma bicarbonate.

Urine

The main features are:

- glycosuria;
- ketonuria.

Management

Urgent medical admission is required. The follow-ing initial blood tests should be carried out, usually by physicians or accident and emergency staff:

- urea and electrolytes (including bicarbonate);
- haemoglobin and haematocrit;
- blood gases;
- acid-base state.
  Management includes:
- administration of insulin – intravenously or intramuscularly;
- intravenous administration of fluid and electro-lytes – sodium chloride intravenous infusion with potassium replacement to prevent insulin – induced hypokalaemia (sodium bicarbonate infu-sion is used only if there is extreme acidosis and shock);
- treatment of any infection.

HYPOGLYCAEMIA IN INSULIN-DEPENDENT DIABETES MELLITUS (IDDM)

Clinical features

The main clinical features of hypoglycaemia in insulin-dependent diabetes mellitus are:

1. history of:
   - excess insulin (excess intake; insulinoma; treatment with a long-acting sulphonylurea, e.g. chlorpropamide or glibenclamide);
   - excess exercise;
   - reduced food intake;
   - large intake of alcohol;
2. rapid onset of symptoms (which may progress to coma);

3. altered behaviour – e.g. aggressive behaviour;
4. raised pulse, systolic blood pressure may be raised;
5. sweating.

Blood

The main feature is hypoglycaemia.

Management

Urgent treatment of the hypoglycaemia is required:

- oral glucose or 3 to 4 lumps of sucrose with a little water, repeated if necessary after 10 to 15 minutes;
- if unconsciousness occurs, intravenously administer up to 50 mL of 50 per cent glucose intravenous infusion.

Glucagon may be administered intramuscularly as an alternative to parenteral glucose.

25

PRACTICAL PROCEDURES

VENEPUNCTURE

The veins commonly accessed are those found in the antecubital fossa, shown in Fig. 25.1.

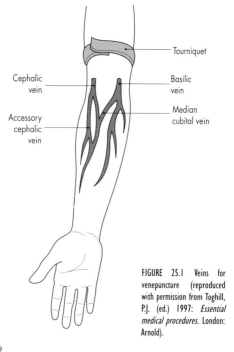

FIGURE 25.1 Veins for venepuncture (reproduced with permission from Toghill, P.J. (ed.) 1997: *Essential medical procedures*. London: Arnold).

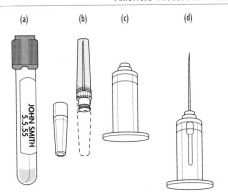

FIGURE 25.2 The apparatus available for the Becton Dickinson Vacutainer system of blood taking. (a) Typical container with rubber diaphragm in the cap. (b) Double-ended needle with green cover protecting bare needle and white/opaque cover protecting rubber-sleeved needle. (c) Needle holder. (d) Needle holder with rubber-sleeved holder screwed into it and green cover removed to expose the bare needle.

It is worth labelling the blood-test bottles in advance. The blood forms vary between different hospitals, and you should be familiar with the ones used locally. Make sure that you know how to use the newer Vacutainer® tubes, with Hemogard™ closure (Becton Dickinson Vacutainer Systems Europe, Meylan, France), shown in Fig. 25.2, if these are used in your hospital or clinic.

Figure 25.3 shows the main steps involved.

MALE URINARY CATHETERIZATION

The indications for this procedure include:
- urinary output monitoring;
- urinary retention – acute or chronic;
- urinary incontinence;
- maintaining bladder drainage postoperatively;
- administering treatment;
- investigations.

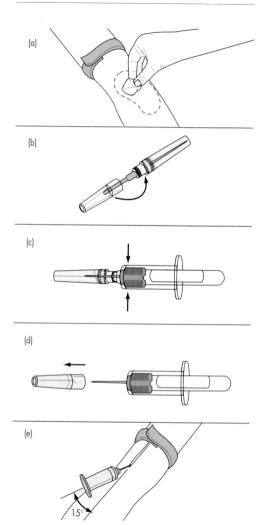

FIGURE 25.3

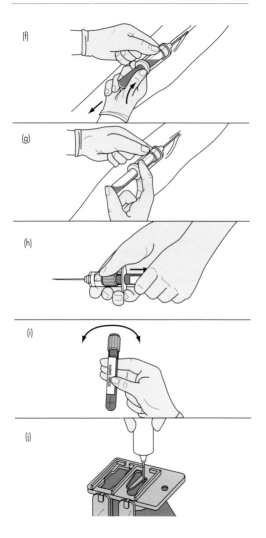

(f)

(g)

(h)

(i)

(j)

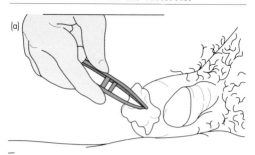

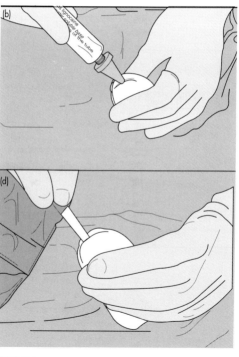

FIGURE 25.4

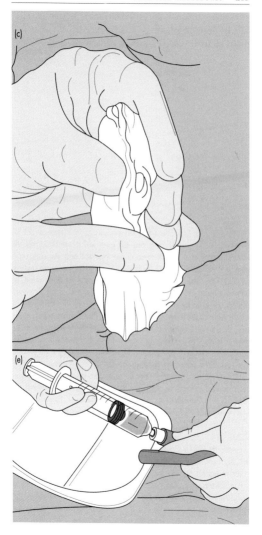

Female urinary catheterization is better carried out by female nursing staff. Figure 25.4 shows the main steps involved in male catheterization.

FIGURE 25.3 The Vacutainer system for venepuncture. (a) Prepare the site for venepuncture. (b) After checking that the paper seal is unbroken, hold the coloured section of the needle-shield in one hand and twist and remove the white section. Discard. (c) Screw the needle into the holder, leaving the coloured shield over the needle. (d) Remove the coloured section of the needle shield. (e) Perform venepuncture in the usual manner with the arm in the downward position. (f) Introduce the tube into the holder; placing the forefinger and middle finger on the flange of the holder and the thumb on the bottom of the tube, push the tube to the end of the holder, puncturing the diaphragm of the stopper. Remove the tourniquet as soon as blood begins to flow into the tube. (g) When the vacuum is exhausted and blood flow ceases, apply a soft pressure with your thumb against the flange to disengage the stopper from the needle. (h) Remove the tube from the holder. Do not remove the needle from the vein until you have removed the (last) tube from the holder. (i) Gently invert the filled tube 8 to 10 times to mix the additives with the blood. Do not shake. (j) Unscrew the used needle and discard it into the Vacutainer disposal box.

FIGURE 25.4 Male catheterization. (a) Cleanse the penis with non-irritant antiseptic. (b) Squeeze Lignocaine jelly (15 mL, 0.5 per cent) down the urethra with one hand, while holding the penis with the other. (c) Squeeze the meatus gently to prevent the jelly from leaking out and then massage it down the urethra towards the perineum. (d) Pulling the penis gently upwards, in order to straighten the urethra, release the pressure on the glans and introduce the catheter into the meatus in the line of the urethra. (e) Continue to pass the catheter until the side arm reaches the meatus. Inflate the balloon with no more than 10 mL of water.

26

INFECTIONS

NOTIFIABLE DISEASES

In the UK, doctors are under a statutory obligation to notify any cases of the following diseases seen by them to the appropriate authority (this information is current at the time of writing and differs in Scotland):

- acute encephalitis;
- acute poliomyelitis;
- anthrax;
- cholera;
- diphtheria;
- dysentery (amoebic or bacillary);
- food poisoning;
- leprosy;
- leptospirosis;
- malaria;
- measles;
- meningitis;
- meningococcal septicaemia (without meningitis);
- mumps;
- ophthalmia neonatorum;
- paratyphoid fever;
- plague;
- rabies;
- relapsing fever;
- rubella;
- scarlet fever;
- smallpox;
- tetanus;

- tuberculosis;
- typhoid fever;
- typhus;
- viral haemorrhagic fever;
- viral hepatitis;
- whooping cough;
- yellow fever.

The local Department of Public Health or Consultant in Communicable Diseases Control should be contacted; their telephone number is available from the local microbiology department. Clinical suspicion is sufficient; a laboratory diagnosis is not required. A fee may be claimed on filling in the appropriate form.

PREVENTION

Factors that may help to prevent and/or control infectious diseases, and which should therefore be considered with regard to psychiatric patients, include:

- immunization;
- good housing and sanitation;
- health education – particularly with respect to sexually transmitted diseases;
- food safety;
- hygiene – wash hands before, between and after examining patients;
- disinfection and sterilization;
- vector control;
- screening;
- tracing of contacts;
- chemoprophylaxis.

NEEDLE-STICK INJURIES

In the event of accidental inoculation with a contaminated 'sharp', such as a used needle, the following procedure should be carried out:

- encourage cuts and needle pricks to bleed;

- wash cuts and needle pricks thoroughly with soap and water;
- cover cuts and needle pricks;
- inform the manager in charge;
- identify the source of the 'sharp';
- obtain a blood sample from the patient by whom the 'sharp' was 'contaminated';
- attend the occupational health department within 1 hour or, if it is closed, attend the accident and emergency department;
- fully complete an accident form as accurately as possible, including details of the source of the 'sharp', and the name, hospital number and ward, or address and telephone number of the patient by whom the 'sharp' was 'contaminated'.

BITE INJURIES

It is possible, in psychiatric practice, to be bitten by a patient. The procedure to be followed in such a case is similar to that given above for needle-stick injuries. It is important to obtain a blood sample from the patient as soon as is practicable. In addition to giving a blood sample yourself, you should also receive a tetanus booster (from occupational health or accident and emergency) if you are not up to date with your tetanus immunization.

Part
V

Management
Issues

27

BED MANAGERS AND EXTRA-CONTRACTUAL REFERRALS

━━━

Pressures on acute psychiatry emergency care in many areas, particularly inner city areas, are heavy and continuous. This puts pressure on community mental health teams, crisis teams and general practitioners together with community psychiatric nurses who support patients in the community with mental health problems. However, the greatest pressure seems to be on in-patient admission facilities, making emergency admissions very difficult. This problem is variable, and it is difficult to identify any single factor that accounts for these increased demands. It seems likely that it is a combination of several different factors, some being more important than others.

- *Demography*: areas with high levels of homelessness, poverty, unemployment and ethnicity tend to have greater psychiatric morbidity.
- *Care in the community*: there are now fewer patients living in long-stay institutions, as a result of the continuing closure of mental hospitals.
- *Breakdown of community services*: the causes can be wide-ranging, from poor compliance with medication to a breakdown in community arrangements such as housing. The patient may have moved from their original catchment area where they are well known to psychiatric services, and so there is no continuity of care.
- *Lack of a mental health crisis response*: The lack of an instant mental health outreach response to a

crisis means that patients will present in a variety of ways. These include the general practitioner, police, social workers or the accident and emergency department. This problem is more severe at weekends.

Alternative factors influencing demand

The accident and emergency department is often the preferred choice of patients, who will present there as it is free from stigma. It can also be designated as a 'place of safety' for Section 136 of the Mental Health Act 1983.

This increased pressure on admissions has led to people spending hours trying to find an empty bed. This situation has resulted in the development of the bed manager. Bed managers are relatively senior clinicians (often nurses), who are responsible for the efficient and effective management of beds in an acute unit. They work in conjunction with ward managers and senior managerial staff Part of their role is also to co-ordinate the out-of-hours bed management rota and the staff involved with it. They also liaise with multiprofessional teams within the area.

Bed managers act as a central resource in problem-solving in relation to waiting lists, referrals and patients waiting for discharge or other in-patient services. They provide regular information to multiprofessional teams and relevant purchasers concerning the day-to-day status of in-patients and those awaiting admission. Sometimes patients are admitted to hospitals that do not fall within the contract of the local purchasers, hence the use of the term extra-contractual referral (ECR). ECRs are often to private psychiatric units; it is the responsibility of the bed manager to keep track of ECRs and to bring the patients back into the referring hospital whenever possible. A substantial number of patients are also in custody or in a regional secure unit, and their admission has to be prioritized.

When the bed manager is not on duty, the duty doctor will often spend substantial amounts of time finding placements for urgent admissions. Problems can also arise when the clarity of nursing and medical roles is blurred.

It is essential that the duty doctor is aware of the overall complexity of the situation and is able to work co-operatively with the bed manager.

28

NATIONAL HEALTH SERVICE MANAGEMENT AND RELATIONSHIPS WITH CLINICIANS

———

The Health Service has gone through many changes since its inception in 1948 when Aneurin Bevan set it up with the aims of equality of service, comprehensive scope, high standards, and to be free at the point of delivery.

In 1983 the Griffiths White Paper conceived the idea that the Health Service would benefit from being run in a similar way to Sainsbury's. Griffiths was the Chairman of Sainsbury's at that time, and he obviously impressed the then Prime Minister, Margaret Thatcher, who asked him to design a new health service. This was the start of the National Health Service Management as we know it. Prior to this there had only been administrators, but now there were District General Managers and a multiplicity of Managers.

In 1990 another White Paper, entitled *Working for People*, was published. This incorporated market forces with purchasers and providers. The providers became Trusts which were run as firms with Chief Executives, Executive Directors and non-Executive Directors who were responsible for budgets. The Trust Board usually has only one doctor and one nurse, and none of the other members are clinically trained. There has been a huge increase in financial staff, with contracts and invoices taking up much time, money and energy.

It is easy to see how economy and solvency have become paramount, with quality of patient care a secondary consideration.

Managers' jobs are insecure, with much competition and tremendous pressure in a system that has not been thought through and which ultimately is not working.

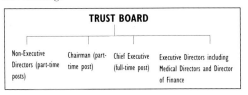

In some Trusts separate areas are managed by clinicians who have a budget and are called Clinical Directors. They usually work part-time clinically, but need an assistant manager if they are not to compromise too much of their clinical work. In other Trusts the clinical input is in the form of a Lead Clinician who does not hold a budget and who is supposed to have a partnership relationship with a manager.

Managers are responsible for monitoring contracts with purchasers.

The contracting process needs to involve clinicians, as does the standard-setting process. Informed clinicians do not need to relinquish control of their affairs to managers, but occasionally maverick managers gain a mistaken sense of their own importance and throw their weight about. It must always be remembered, however, that patients do not attend to see managers but to be treated by clinicians.

A few more changes of government and structure of the Health Service may see the end of management as we know it, but clinicians will still be needed.

Part
VI

Looking
After
Yourself

29

YOUR CAREER

▬

The following points apply particularly to those who wish to pursue a career in psychiatry. However, many of the points are also relevant to those in a psychiatric post as part of their training for another speciality, such as medicine or general practice.

Clinical experience

- Try to gain supervised clinical experience in different clinical psychiatric specialties; this is also helpful in terms of professional examinations such as the MRCPsych.
- On-call work and ward-round presentations provide useful learning experiences and excellent preparation for the clinical parts of the MRCPsych examination.

Course attendance

- Ensure that you attend a course of theoretical instruction such as the 3-year courses recommended as part of UK training.
- You should also regularly attend journal clubs, reading seminars and guest lectures; in addition to forming an important part of your training, such attendance can be helpful in preparing for the MRCPsych examination and also helps to develop your capacity to evaluate published research critically.

MRCPsych examination

- Begin your preparation for each part of this examination as early as possible.
- Practise presenting cases to senior colleagues; if possible, use video feedback occasionally.

- Set yourself a realistic revision timetable (with time built in for unexpected events, such as illness), and stick to it.
- Ensure that you are familiar with the contents of good standard textbooks and test yourself regularly; the questions in revision books are often worth attempting.
- If you are worried about your knowledge close to the examination, it may be worth attending a short revision course; however, this may not be necessary if you have worked diligently throughout your training.
- Ensure that you are familiar with the current structure of the examination; obtain details of this, the curriculum, specimen papers and past papers at an early stage in your examination preparation.
- Attempt specimen and past papers under examination conditions; practise similarly for the clinical components of the examination.

Career pathways
- Seek advice from your tutor/educational supervisor and the consultants for whom you work throughout your training.
- The latest advice on training should be read; at the time of writing, in the UK this is *A Guide to Specialist Registrar Training*, (also known as the 'Orange Guide') published by the Department of Health in March 1996.
- Figure 29.1 summarizes the UK career pathways for higher specialist trainees undertaking research (NTN = National Training Number; CCST = Certificate of Completion of Specialist Training; SpR = specialist registrar); this figure is based on a supplement to the 'Orange Guide'.

Research publications
- If you wish to publish research in order to enhance your curriculum vitae, but you do not intend to pursue a career in research, then

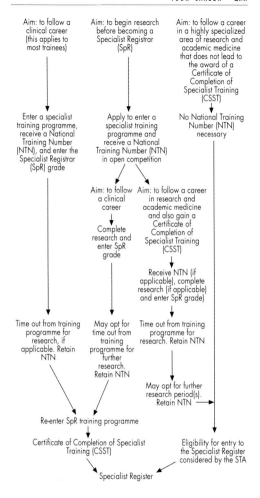

FIGURE 29.1 Career pathways for higher specialist trainees undertaking research (based on *Academic and Research Medicine: Supplement to a Guide to Specialist Registrar Training (March 1996)* London: Department of Health).

obtain advice from your tutor or educational supervisor and consider approaching someone who is actively involved in research in an area that interests you.

- It may be worth considering starting by writing up a short case report of interest, or a small study.

Job interviews

- Ask a senior colleague to look over your curriculum vitae.
- Rehearse your interview technique with someone senior; video feedback is often helpful.

30

YOUR TUTOR–SUPERVISOR

The Royal College of Psychiatrists has been very responsible in its training role for a considerable time, and well-organized training schemes function up and down the country. They are regularly and rigorously inspected and approval is removed or only given temporarily if they do not come up to the required standard.

Since the reorganization following the Calman Report, this is now complemented by the Postgraduate Dean's Office, which should work in tandem with the College training rules, although some streamlining is still required, and the number of visits seems to have doubled, which is probably unnecessary.

Categories of tutors

Category 1 – Psychiatric Tutor – Unit Tutor in Psychiatry

This post is filled by a psychiatrist working in the unit, and most consultants occupy the post at some time in their career. It sometimes seems that each additional consultant quickly becomes the tutor.

These tutors are responsible for the day-to-day running of the training, and have a responsibility to ensure that the Postgraduate Medical Education Programme is implemented. They may be responsible for educational equipment such as projectors and video cameras, and they must ensure that a library with all the necessary facilities is available. This may be situated in a local Postgraduate Centre, or it may be in the local medical school library. The tutors have responsibility for supervision of their local trainees in conjunction with the rotation tutor.

It is the local tutor's responsibility to ensure that everything meets the necessary standard, from the on-call room to supervision of trainees by trainers.

Local tutors also usually deal with examination candidates who are experiencing difficulties or who merely need encouragement.

Category 2 – Rotation Tutor – Co-ordinating Tutor
This is a psychiatrist responsible for co-ordinating a large training scheme at a regional level, who may work with other rotational tutors. He or she may be the college tutor at his or her own hospital, and will participate in a training committee and encourage junior doctors to be representatives on the committee. The rotational tutor will meet each trainee on a regular basis and will be involved with the college tutor if a trainee has a particularly difficult problem.

Category 3 – Scheme Organizer
This is a demanding role for a psychiatrist, and the scheme organizer needs a recognised session in which to carry out the organization.

The scheme organizer co-ordinates a large training scheme, sometimes with as many as 90 trainees, and has to ensure that each trainee has a satisfactory range of experience. He or she also has to make sure that the Training Committee is aware of all college policy on training matters, and of all relevant documents.

It is important that the Training Committee, which is a college structure, remains independent and does not simply execute the policies of the Postgraduate Dean.

A trainee in any rotational scheme should meet regularly with his or her psychiatric tutor, and any problems which he or she encounters in training will benefit from an airing with the tutor.

Supervision of trainees by trainers

The timetabled hour each week is intended to enable the trainee to receive feedback about his or her performance and to discuss any training difficulties, as well as academic or career problems.

It has the added advantage that it improves the working relationship between the trainee and trainer and, if working well, it will provide support for both participants.

Some trainees are reluctant to participate in supervision, perhaps because they perceive it as threatening. Similarly, some trainers do not feel comfortable with supervision, and will cancel sessions at the first opportunity.

31

ASKING FOR ADVICE

SOURCES OF ADVICE

These include:
- nurses;
- other colleagues;
- senior colleagues;
- consultant on call;
- manager on call.

Junior Doctors are frequently the front-line person at times when there is little support around and, as the least experienced person, they make decisions alone at the most risky moments. Patients may not be admitted or given the appropriate response, and they then have to return home in the middle of the night with the situation unchanged. They may still want to harm themselves or others. However, it is not possible to admit everyone on request, nor is it possible to provide adequate community support, so such decisions sometimes have to be made.

A culture has evolved whereby individuals try to carry on doing this work on their own, and it is perceived as weakness to consult with others too often. It is important for the person in question, when he or she is feeling lonely and under pressure, to remember sources of help such as the following.

- Experienced nurses may well know the people concerned and have seen the situation before and, if asked, will usually give an opinion.

- Other colleagues will be willing both to engage in discussion of the subject, which can clarify thinking, and to offer objective opinions.
- Depending on the rota, sometimes another senior colleague as well as a consultant on call will be available. They are there to be consulted, and it is better to call them in a crisis than for the senior on call to have to pick up the pieces the next day.
- In certain situations the manager on call can help with problems concerning bed shortages, hospital environmental problems and security.

Sometimes senior staff on call do not react well to being called and are not consistently supportive. In this situation it may be possible to contact another more supportive person who is not on call, and to discuss the matter with your tutor as soon as possible.

32

EMOTIONAL SUPPORT AND DEALING WITH STRESS

No medical career is without stress; each has its pressures and rewards. Often a degree of stress can give an edge to work; and some people perform better while under stress. However, excessive stress can be detrimental, and working with people with mental health problems in today's National Health Service often means that there is too much stress.

Research has shown that up to 50 per cent of Junior Doctors, Senior Doctors and Health Service Managers are stressed, and about half of this number scored for depression.

Mental health work gives rise to two forms of stress. The first is due to the actual problems with which the patient presents and the impact these have on the individual at that moment in time. An out-patient clinic, with its typical variety and complexity of patients' problems, can leave the mental health workers feeling emotionally exhausted. Secondly, stress arises from dealing with disorders that do not pursue a straightforward course towards cure. Patients are people first and foremost, but their disorder also has to be diagnosed and their symptoms categorized into prognostic significance. R. D. Laing pointed out that individuals often protect themselves from the distress of others by the mechanism of objectification.

Perhaps it is more helpful to alternate between identification with and observation of the patient.

The organization of the service in which the patients and staff find themselves can also contribute to stress. Ideally, the service providers should be concerned about patient need and how best to provide it. This can be difficult at the best of times, but in today's National Health Service, which changes frequently and is unduly politicized, the public service philosophy has given way to a phoney market-place philosophy. One example of the adverse effects of putting market forces before quality of care for patients is that general practitioners may prescribe outdated and relatively unsafe tricyclic antidepressants rather than safer but more expensive newer antidepressants.

The managers are under pressure to meet their demands in this system, and have to carry with them clinicians whose training and practice are at variance with today's Health Service. This leads to problems and confrontations, with each group neither appreciating nor understanding the demands being made on the other.

In addition to the pressures outlined above there are many other sources of stress, such as long hours, work overload, job insecurity, harassment, family problems, etc.

Junior Doctors are to some extent protected from the doctor–manager conflict, and have a system of supervision and training which is monitored and protected, and a dedicated tutor.

They also have the support of each other and, where the firms are not disrupted by shift work, they benefit from a support structure which is in some ways similar to a family.

Most Junior Doctors are quite sensible about getting exercise and fresh air and maintaining outside interests. Increasing numbers have access to psychotherapy training and even staff support groups.

33

SERIOUS PROFESSIONAL
MISCONDUCT

The GMC, which is the governing body of doctors, is composed of 50 members. Of these, 34 doctors are selected by Universities and Royal Colleges and nine are nominated (these are usually lay people).

The GMC controls medical education and maintains a register of qualified practitioners. It also provides advice for doctors on standards of professional conduct and medical ethics.

The GMC is required to set up a Health Committee which deals with doctors who may be unfit to practise because of physical or mental illness.

The Professional Conduct Committee is able to discipline any doctor who has committed an offence or is guilty of serious professional misconduct.

Discipline may mean that the doctor is removed from the register, or he or she may be suspended for a year or have to retrain or attend a course.

Earlier legislation defined punishable professional misconduct, which today is defined as 'conduct . . .reasonably regarded as dishonourable by professional brethren of good repute and competency'.

Thus adultery with a patient or a patient's spouse is still regarded as serious misconduct, and drug and alcohol abuse and fraud have joined the list, as well as touting for custom. The charge must be proved beyond all reasonable doubt, as the doctor can lose his or her career as a result.

If dissatisfied with a verdict, a doctor may appeal to the Privy Council. The evidence will then be reconsidered.

Any doctor who is found guilty of a crime in court (other than a minor driving offence) will automatically have his or her conviction brought in front of the GMC.

The impaired physician

The *American College of Physicians Ethics Manual* states that 'Every physician is responsible for protecting patients from an impaired physician and assisting a Colleague whose professional capability is impaired'.

Impairment may occur because of psychiatric or medical disorders such as HIV infection or the use of mind-altering and habit-forming drugs, e.g. alcohol or heroin. Organic illness may also interfere with cognitive and motor skills, e.g. Alzheimer's disease and Parkinson's disease. Although there is no statement such as the above which pertains to UK doctors, the ethical responsibility must remain universal. However, UK doctors are rather ineffective in doing anything about a colleague's impairment, and tend to shelter behind the Hippocratic Oath.

The system which previously used to exist, consisting of Three Wise Persons (male and female), is less used now since the advent of Trusts, but similar types of organization are utilized, with senior doctors being responsible for individuals who will not accept responsibility for themselves. This applies particularly to doctors affected by substance misuse or mental illness, and not to those who seek appropriate treatment and advice for their problems and who adhere to that advice.

Part VIII

Useful Addresses for Doctors, Patients and Relatives

34

KEEPING RECORDS OF PSYCHIATRIC CARE

Medical records are prepared and maintained by medical record departments. They have a duty to maintain these records so long as the patient is alive, and they cannot destroy them for 20 years after the patient's death, although they are often transferred to microfile.

Records can be single medical records, but in psychiatry multidisciplinary records are now becoming more common, rather than having a separate record for each discipline. The outside cover will usually say 'CONFIDENTIAL – NOT TO BE SEEN BY PATIENT', but patients can now ask for and obtain permission to read their records.

The front cover will state the hospital and Trust that are caring for the patient and the front page will include demographic details. This is usually followed by a space for handwritten records, and then there is a space for correspondence and investigations.

In psychiatry, Care Programme Approach forms are included, and an up-to-date care plan should be available.

Each time any clinician has contact with a patient or their carers, an entry should be made (dated, legible and signed) stating the situation concerning that intervention, the patient's mental state, physical state, medication, etc.

The notes should be written and arranged in sequence, and should not be interfered with subsequently. They form a record.

35

PROCEDURE AFTER A DEATH SUSPECTED AS RESULTING FROM SUICIDE

———

Notification

Clinical staff

The relevant RMO should be informed, as should other medical, nursing and paramedical staff who have been involved with the patient.

Manager

The appropriate manager or managers should be informed and given a brief summary of the patient's history and events. In the event of clinical involvement of Trusts, e.g. a Mental Health Trust using another Trust's hotel facilities, both sets of managers should be involved as the press, etc., do not necessarily know this.

Police and coroner

The police and coroner should be involved and the body should not be moved until the arrival of the police. This should not interfere with resuscitation attempts.

Next of kin

The next of kin should be informed as soon as possible and in as sensitive a way as possible. The best approach is to visit at home, but this is not always possible. Someone who knows the next of kin as well as the deceased should do this task. The breaking of bad news by telephone requires special skills, and messages should never be left on answer machines.

General practitioner
The general practitioner will have a role in supporting the family, and therefore needs to be informed as soon as possible.

Debriefing

Staff and patients
Senior clinical staff should convene a meeting of staff and also of patients as soon as possible to allow ventilation of feelings in response to the patient's death. Some staff should be seen individually.

Next of kin and other relatives
These should be seen as soon as possible by the consultant before psychological barriers are created. Anger towards hospital staff is very common.

Media contact
This is best left to senior management staff, and enquiries should be tactfully channelled towards them.

Continued support is often not available. There will be the ordeal of the Coroner's Court, when key people will have to give evidence so that the coroner can decide on the facts leading to the patient's death. It is important that no member of staff attends the Coroner's Court alone and unsupported. Hospital solicitors and, if necessary, a barrister should be available.

Serious incident inquiries are now the order of the day and can be very stressful. Further debriefing is recommended, but the previous ordeals often do not help to get the whole trauma into perspective for staff and the family, who will need further meetings and support.

They form a record which is sometimes needed for the Coroner's Court, Civil Court, or for the patient to read.

36

CORONER'S COURT

The Coroner's Court is presided over by the Coroner, who is often dually qualified as both a lawyer and a doctor. The court's purpose is to investigate the circumstances of death of a person for whom no death certificate can be written.

This usually includes people who have died as a result of an accident or self-harm, an operation or any situation where the cause of death was unclear and the attending physician is unable to enlighten people further. The Coroner's assistants will collect information from all the people involved with the deceased prior to death, and will usually have a pathologist carry out a post-mortem.

When all of the information has been collected, an inquest will be called and all individuals involved will be summoned to give evidence under oath.

A member of the local press is usually present and records all of the proceedings, unless the inquest is of national interest, when other reporters will be present.

There may be an adversarial situation in which the family of the deceased may feel that a particular aspect of the deceased's care was not adequate or appropriate, and will wish to make this point.

If summoned to the Coroner's Court, it is important to obtain as much information as possible about the deceased, and to go prepared to give evidence after writing a report. It may be that a patient committed suicide after being seen by you in Casualty, or after he or she left the ward. The hospital or Trust may be aware of the family's concern and have a barrister in court.

It is important not to attend the Coroner's Court on your own, but to take support, as the procedure can be very stressful. The Coroner may not understand your position in the hospital and expect a broader knowledge and responsibility than you have.

37

DEALING WITH THE PRESS

It is difficult to maintain an approach which recognizes the interests of the press and broadcasting media, as the work of the public organization, while at the same time protecting patient confidentiality. It is important to maintain good relations between the press and yourself, but your overriding responsibility is to protect the confidential relationship between yourself and your patient. Information of a personal nature should never be disclosed without the patient's consent. The fact that a patient is being seen by a psychiatrist should not be disclosed, and Junior Doctors who are not used to the tenacity of journalists should beware of inadvertently divulging such information.

It is always advisable to ascertain who handles press inquiries in the area where you are employed. There is often a specific *press officer* who is skilled in dealing with press members, and he or she should be briefed accordingly.

When your patient places information with the press, the constraints of confidentiality no longer apply and your Trust can respond to comments or criticisms, but is restricted to the facts. In cases where a well-known figure is known to be in the care of a psychiatrist, and information has been leaked out, a senior member of the Trust may have to make a public statement.

38

COMPETENCY

1. The patient must communicate a choice.
2. The patient must be able to understand relevant information about the proposed medical treatment and treatment alternatives.
3. The patient must be able to appreciate his or her clinical situation.
4. The patient must be able to manipulate information rationally. When someone is incompetent, others have to make decisions for them in a way that takes into account that person's values and expressed wishes. Decisions also have to be made in such a way as to be in the patient's best interests.

39

COURT OF PROTECTION

The Court of Protection is an office of the Supreme Court in the UK which manages the property and affairs of people with mental health problems who are incapable of managing their own affairs. There is also an emergency power (Section 98 of the Act) to protect the property of someone who may later be declared incapable.

Applications

Applications are usually made to the Court by solicitors, local authority receivership departments, and sometimes by relatives. This is done by written application (Form CPI), and is accompanied by a medical certificate (Form CP3) and a fee.

Medical certificate

Only one certificate is required from a registered medical practitioner who has examined the patient. This is usually the patient's general practitioner or a psychiatrist, but the examination is not necessarily carried out by a person who is able to assess the patient's capacity to handle their own affairs.

Of the court's cases, 82 per cent are over 55 years of age, and the majority are women suffering from senile dementia, but the Court does not use advisers who are appropriately trained in Psychiatry of Old Age.

The Royal College of Psychiatrists and the British Medical Association have issued notes of guidance to accompany Form CP3.

Receivership

The Court, if it accepts the incapacity of the patient, will appoint someone to manage the patient's affairs on his or her behalf. This person is called the *receiver*.

Receivers are usually relatives, friends, or solicitors, accountants or bank managers. If no suitable receiver is available, The Court will appoint a Public Trustee. Receivership is monitored by the Court through the Receivership Division of the Public Trust Office, and concerns about the receiver abusing his or her powers should be addressed immediately to them. A receiver is obliged to use the patient's money for that person's benefit. There is a substantial financial implication if a patient has come under the Court of Protection, as the administrative costs have to be paid for, and there is a tendency for safety in investments, rather than profit. The assets of the patient would normally exceed £8000 before it became feasible for their affairs to be managed by the Court. Should the patient be incapable of making a will, the Court will draw up a statutory will which is well researched and sensitively constructed. The Court is a safeguard when financial abuse is suspected and the patient is incapable of managing his or her affairs. However, in the event of a dispute over the degree of incapacity there does not appear to be any appeal procedure and, as previously mentioned, medical advisers are not necessarily qualified in the appropriate specialty.

40

POWER OF ATTORNEY AND ENDURING POWER OF ATTORNEY

Power of Attorney is a legal device for agency whereby the person involved allows one or several others to act for him or her in a limited or un-limited capacity in matters relating to finances and property.

The ordinary Power of Attorney becomes invalid as soon as the patient becomes incapable of managing his or her affairs.

There is frequent misuse of this form of delegation, with solicitors and family indicating that the patient signed it in a lucid moment.

In 1986, the Enduring Power of Attorney was introduced to provide for those who later became incapable through mental disorder of managing their affairs. The Enduring Power of Attorney (EPA) can only be signed when the patient is still capable of managing his or her affairs, although there is some flexibility in this. The EPA must be registered with the GP when the person becomes incapable, and there is no monitoring of the attorney's performance. It may be arranged so that the patient continues to manage their own affairs until they become incapable.

An EPA does not confer the power to influence medical treatment.

The idea is that the patient can make up their own mind as to who will manage their affairs should they become incapable, rather than have the Court of Protection decide, and obviously it will cost less in the right hands, but there is great potential for abuse.

41

MEDICAL TREATMENT UNDER COMMON LAW

Every adult has the right to decide if he or she will accept medical treatment, even if refusal will lead to irreparable damage or even death, so long as he or she has the capacity to decide. It does not matter whether the reasons for refusal are rational or irrational. The general attitude is always to preserve the life and health of everyone, and this may seem to go against this basic belief. However, not everyone has the capacity to make such decisions.

An otherwise capable person may be temporarily deprived of his or her capacity by the effects of fatigue, shock, pain, drugs or unconsciousness. They may also be deprived of this ability by long-term mental incapacity such as Alzheimer's disease or retarded development. If the patient does not have the capacity to decide at the time of refusal, and continues to be incapable, it is the duty of the doctors to treat that patient according to his or her best interests. For example, on an orthopaedic ward it is not uncommon for elderly patients with fractured femurs, and who are also suffering from senile dementia, to deny their fractures and refuse consent to treatment. Clearly it is in their best interests to have their fractures surgically repaired, for if they were left untreated this would lead to serious damage to health, if not death.

If a patient refuses to give consent, careful consideration of his or her capacity is needed. It may be a straightforward question of capacity or no capacity, but the patient may have reduced capacity. The question therefore is whether the capacity is reduced below the level needed in a case of this importance. Refusals are not all equally significant. Some may result in serious consequences, while others may not. Undue influence may be brought to bear on the patient by his or her spouse, parents or religious adviser. Some relationships more readily lend themselves to exerting pressure to the extent of influencing the person to make a decision that he or she would not otherwise have made. For example, a dominant daughter who has continually threatened her frail mother with physical abuse may render the mother unable to make satisfactory independent decisions, through fear and habituation.

Doctors always need to ask themselves why the patient has refused treatment. Are the present circumstances those which one would expect, or are his or her decisions based on a false assumption?

Doctors should not hesitate to seek the advice of the courts in a situation where the patient's life is threatened by their refusal of treatment.

42

FITNESS TO DRIVE

The right to drive a car is not regarded as a basic human right, but is viewed in much the same way as the right to use a gun, for obvious reasons. There is evidence that older drivers who are involved in road traffic accidents are more likely to be killed or seriously injured than younger drivers. Oxley demonstrated an 80 per cent increase in fatalities and an increase of 144 per cent of all highway accidents in individuals aged 70 years or over, for the period 1981–1990.

Older people often have not taken a driving test, and the volume of traffic has increased and road layout has become more complex during their driving career. They may also have poor vision, or be taking medication with side-effects, as well as having practical driving-skill problems. People often continue to drive in the early stages of a dementing illness, and it is difficult to know when they should stop. The responsibility for removing the licence lies with the Drivers and Vehicle Licensing Authority (DVLA). The patient's doctor should encourage the patient to report their problems to the DVLA, but if they do not have sufficient insight or choose not to do so, the patient's doctor may approach the doctor at the DVLA, who is experienced in dealing with these problems and will obtain a second opinion before making a decision.

People with serious mental illness should inform the DVLA of their condition, as should people with epilepsy, diabetes, etc., and a questionnaire will be sent to their doctor or psychiatrist to be completed.

Should they be judged safe to drive, this licence will only extend for 3 years and will be reviewed again after that period.

The address for the DVLA Medical Advisory Branch is as follows:

Department of Transport
Medical Advisory Branch
Oldway Centre
Orchard Street
Swansea SA1 ITU
Tel: 01792 304 747

43

MENTAL HEALTH LEGISLATION

ENGLAND AND WALES: MENTAL HEALTH ACT 1983

Section 1: definitions

Mental disorder
Mental illness, arrested or incomplete development of mind, psychopathic disorder and any other disorder or disability of mind.

Severe mental impairment
A state of arrested or incomplete development of mind which includes severe impairment of intelligence and social functioning and is associated with abnormally aggressive or seriously irresponsible conduct on the part of the person concerned.

Mental impairment
A state of arrested or incomplete development of mind (not amounting to severe mental impairment) which includes significant impairment of intelligence and social functioning and is associated with abnormally aggressive or seriously irresponsible conduct on the part of the person concerned.

Psychopathic disorder
A persistent disorder or disability of mind (whether or not this includes significant impairment of intelligence) which results in abnormally aggressive or seriously irresponsible conduct on the part of the person concerned.

Patient
A person suffering from or appearing to suffer from mental disorder.

Medical treatment
Includes nursing, and care and rehabilitation under medical supervision.

Responsible Medical Officer (RMO)
The registered medical practitioner in charge of the treatment of the patient, that is, the consultant psychiatrist, or, if he or she is not available, the doctor who for the time being is in charge of the patient's treatment may deputize.

Approved Doctor
A registered medical practitioner approved under Section 12 of the Act by the Secretary of State (with authority being delegated to the Regional Health Authority) as having special experience in the diagnosis or treatment of mental disorder.

Approved Social Worker (ASW)
An officer of a local social services authority with appropriate training who may make applications for compulsory admission; hospital senior social workers usually hold lists of Approved Social Workers.

Nearest relative
The first surviving person living in the UK in the following list, with full blood relatives taking preference over half blood relatives, and the elder of two relatives of the same description or level of kinship also taking preference:
1. husband or wife;
2. son or daughter;
3. father or mother;
4. brother or sister;
5. grandparent;
6. grandchild;
7. uncle or aunt;
8. nephew or niece.

Preference is also given to a relative with whom the patient ordinarily lives, or by whom he or she is cared for.

Note that the term *mental illness* is not formally defined; its operational definition is a matter of clinical judgement in each case. The Act states that a person may *not* be dealt with under the Mental Health Act as suffering from *mental disorder* 'by reason only of promiscuity or other immoral conduct, sexual deviancy or dependence on alcohol or drugs'.

Civil treatment orders

Table 43.1 shows the civil treatment orders under the Mental Health Act 1983.

Supervision registers

The three categories of risk for inclusion on a supervision register are that a patient should be at:

- significant risk of suicide and/or;
- significant risk of serious violence to others and/or;
- significant risk of severe self-neglect.

The decision to include a patient on a supervision register is made by the RMO in consultation with the multidisciplinary team (*see also* The Role of the Responsible Medical Officer, pp.10–14).

Consent to treatment

Table 43.2 shows consent to treatment under the Mental Health Act 1983. Such consent should be informed and voluntary, implying that mental illness, such as dementia, does not affect the patient's judgement.

Forensic treatment orders

Table 43.3 shows forensic treatment orders for mentally abnormal offenders.

MENTAL HEALTH (SCOTLAND) ACT 1984

Table 43.4 sets out equivalent Scottish and English Mental Health Act treatment orders.

TABLE 43.1 Civil treatment order under the Mental Health Act 1983 (reproduced with permission from Puri, B.K., Laking, P.J. and Treasaden, I.H. 1996: *Textbook of psychiatry*. Edinburgh: Churchill Livingstone)

Civil treatment order under Mental Health Act 1983	Grounds	Application by	Medical recommendations	Maximum duration	Eligibility for appeal to Mental Health Review Tribunal
Section 2 Admission for assessment	Mental disorder	Nearest relative or approved social worker	Two doctors (one approved under Section 12)	28 days	Within 14 days
Section 3 Admission for treatment	Mental illness, psychopathic disorder, mental impairment, severe mental impairment (If psychopathic disorder or mental impairment, treatment must be likely to alleviate or prevent deterioration)	Nearest relative or approved social worker	Two doctors (one approved under Section 12)	6 months	Within first 6 months. If renewed, within second 6 months, then every year. Mandatory every 3 years
Section 4 Emergency admission for assessment	Mental disorder (urgent necessity)	Nearest relative or approved social worker	Any doctor	72 hours	

Section	Condition	Applied by	Notes	Duration
Section 5(2) Urgent detention of voluntary in-patient	Danger to self or to others	Doctor in charge of patient's care		72 hours
Section 5(4) Nurses holding power of voluntary in-patient	Mental disorder (danger to self, health or others)	Registered mental nurse or registered nurse for mental handicap	None	6 hours
Section 136 Admission by police	Mental disorder	Police officer	Allows patient in public place to be removed to 'place of safety'	72 hours
Section 135	Mental disorder	Magistrates	Allows power of entry to home and removal of patient to place of safety	72 hours

TABLE 43.3 Forensic treatment orders for mentally abnormal offenders (reproduced with permission from Puri, B.K., Laking, P.J. and Treasaden, I.H. 1996: *Textbook of psychiatry*. Edinburgh: Churchill Livingstone)

	Grounds	Made by	Medical recommendations	Maximum duration	Eligibility for appeal to Mental Health Review Tribunal
Section 35 Remand to hospital for report	Mental disorder	Magistrates or Crown Court	Any doctor	28 days. Renewable at 28-day intervals. Maximum 12 weeks	
Section 36 Remand to hospital for treatment	Mental illness, severe mental impairment (*not if charged with murder*)	Crown Court	Two doctors: one approved under Section 12	28 days. Renewable at 28-days intervals. Maximum 12 weeks	
Section 37 Hospital and guardianship orders	Mental disorder. (If psychopathic disorder or mental impairment must be likely to alleviate or prevent deterioration.) Accused of, or convicted for, an imprisonable offence	Magistrates or Crown Court	Two doctors, one approved under Section 12	6 months. Renewable for further 6 months and then annually	During second 6 months. Then every year. Mandatory every 3 years

Section					
Section 41 Restriction order	Added to Section 37. To protect public from serious harm	Crown Court	Oral evidence from one doctor	Usually without limit of time. Effect: leave, transfer, or discharge only with consent of Home Secretary	As Section 37
Section 38 Interim hospital order	Mental disorder For trial of treatment	Magistrates or Crown Court	Two doctors: one approved under Section 12	12 weeks. Renewable at 28-day intervals Maximum 6 months	None
Section 47 Transfer of a sentenced prisoner to hospital	Mental disorder	Home Secretary	Two doctors: one approved under Section 12	Until earliest date of release from sentence	Once in the first 6 months. Then once in the next 6 months. Thereafter, once a year
Section 48 Urgent transfer to hospital of remand prisoner	Mental disorder	Home Secretary	Two doctors: one approved under Section 12	Until date of trial	Once in the first 6 months. Then once in the next 6 months. Thereafter, once a year
Section 49 Restriction direction	Added to Section 47 or Section 48	Home Secretary	—	Until end of Section 47 or 48. Effect: leave, transfer or discharge only with consent of Home Secretary	As for Section 47 and 48 to which applied

TABLE 43.2 Consent to treatment under the Mental Health Act 1983 (reproduced with permission from Puri, B.K., Laking, P.J. and Treasaden, I.H. 1996: *Textbook of psychiatry.* Edinburgh: Churchill Livingstone)

Type of treatment	Informal	Detained
Urgent treatment	No consent	No consent
Section 57 Irreversible, hazardous or non-established treatments, e.g. psychosurgery (e.g. leucotomy), hormone implants (for sex offenders), surgical operations (e.g. castration)	Consent and second opinion	Consent and second opinion
Section 58 Psychiatric drugs, ECT	Consent	Consent or second opinion

1. For first 3 months of treatment a detained patient's consent is not required for Section 58 medicines, but is for ECT.
2. Patients can withdraw voluntary consent at any time.

GUARDIANSHIP (MENTAL HEALTH ACT 1983)

The purpose of guardianship is to enable a small number of mentally disordered people who do not require treatment in hospital, either formally or informally, but who need close supervision and some control in the community, as a consequence of their mental disorder, to receive community care. These people include individuals who are able to cope provided that they take their medication regularly, but who fail to do so. Also included are those who neglect themselves to the point of seriously endangering their health. Thus the purpose is to ensure that patients receive community care where it cannot be otherwise provided without compulsion. It enables the patient to live as independently as possible. Under the Mental Health Act 1983 a guardianship order may be made in respect of a patient over 16 years of age, on the grounds that he or she is suffering from a mental disorder of a nature or degree that warrants his or her reception into guardianship.

TABLE 43.4 Equivalent Scottish and English Mental Health Act treatment orders (reproduced with permission from Puri, B.K., Laking, P.J. and Treasaden, I.H. 1996: *Textbook of psychiatry*. Edinburgh: Churchill Livingstone)

Treatment Order	Mental Health (England & Wales) Act 1983	Mental Health (Scotland) 1984
Emergency admission	Section 4	Section 24
Short-term detention	Section 2	Section 26
Admission for treatment	Section 3	Section 22
Nurses holding power of a voluntary in-patient	Section 5(4) (for 6 hours)	Section 25(2) for 2 hrs
Guardianship	Section 37	Section 37
Committal to hospital pending trial	Section 36	Sections 25 & 330 of the 1975 Act
Remand for enquiry into mental condition	Section 35	Sections 180 & 381 of the 1975 Act
Removal to hospital of persons in prison awaiting trial or sentence	Section 48	Section 70
Interim hospital order	Section 38	Sections 174a & 375a of the 1975 Act amended by the Mental Health (Amendment) (Scotland) Act 1983
Hospital order	Section 37	Sections 175 & 376 of the 1975 Act
Restriction order	Section 41	Sections 178 & 379 by the 1975 Act
Transfer of prisoner under sentence to hospital	Section 47	Section 71

An application may be made more usually by Social Services, but provision does exist for the nearest relative to do this. The designated guardian is usually the director of the local Social Services – hence the use of guardianship has declined. It is not used at all in some places.

Powers of guardianship

The patient is required:

- to live at a given address as specified by the guardian;
- to attend at specified places, e.g. out-patient clinics, for medical treatment;
- to give access at any place of residence to an approved social worker or other specified person.

It does not give the right to transport the patient to the given address, and it does not give the right to insist on taking medication.

Supervision

(See Discharge Planning and Community Care, pp. 169–71.)

44

TRIBUNALS

Under the Mental Health Act 1983, Mental Health Review Tribunals are independent bodies allowing patients who are detained under this Act to have a review carried out of this detention, and allowing a right of appeal by patients who do not wish to continue to be detained compulsorily in hospital or be compulsorily under guardianship. The minimum membership of a Mental Health Review Tribunal is:

- a legal member – who is the President of the Mental Health Review Tribunal;
- a medical member – usually a consultant psychiatrist;
- a lay member.

During their training, psychiatry trainees should ensure that they attend Mental Health Review Tribunals, with permission, in order to gain practical experience of the workings of these bodies. According to the Code of Practice (1990):

There is a statutory obligation on the Managers to tell a detained patient of his right to apply to a Mental Health Review Tribunal. In addition, Managers should regard it as an obligation to ensure that patients and their nearest relatives know of the existence and role of these tribunals and of their respective rights of application to them. The Managers should ensure that patients remain aware of their rights to apply to a tribunal and are given every opportunity and assistance to exercise those rights, including facilities for representation. The patient should be told of his right to be represented by a lawyer of his choice, the Law Society's Mental Health Review Tribunal representation panel list and about other appropriate organisations, and should be given every assistance in using any of them. Managers should designate a member of staff to see personally every detained patient who applies to a tribunal or who is referred to a tribunal and to give them every reasonable assistance in securing representation (if the patient wishes).

Patients or their nearest relatives in the following categories may apply to a Mental Health Review Tribunal:

- a patient detained under Section 2 may apply within 14 days of admission;
- a patient detained under Section 3 may apply within 6 months of admission;
- a patient received into guardianship under Section 7 may apply within 6 months of the date of the order;
- a patient or nearest relative may apply within 28 days of the date they were informed of the patient's Mental Health Act diagnostic reclassification (Section 16);
- a patient transferred from guardianship to hospital under Section 19 may apply within 6 months of the transfer;
- a patient who is detained in hospital for treatment or who is subject to guardianship may apply to a Mental Health Review Tribunal within each period following renewal of the order (first 6 months following renewal, then during each subsequent 12-month period) (Section 20);
- the nearest relative of a patient detained for treatment who has requested the discharge of the patient may apply within 28 days of being told that a report of the Responsible Medical Officer prevents the discharge (Section 25);
- when a nearest relative of a patient detained in hospital or subject to a guardianship order has had their authority removed by a County Court order, they may apply to a Mental Health Review Tribunal once every 12 months (Section 29).

In addition to deciding whether or not to direct the discharge of a patient, other choices available to a Mental Health Review Tribunal include recommending that a patient be granted leave of absence, be transferred to another hospital, or be transferred into guardianship.

The Mental Health Review Tribunal has to make decisions on the patient's care on the following legal grounds:

Decision of Tribunal

1. Is the Tribunal satisfied that the patient is not now suffering from mental illness, psychopathic disorder, severe mental impairment or mental impairment, or from any of those forms of disorder of a nature or degree which makes it appropriate for the patient to be liable to be detained in a hospital for medical treatment?   Yes/No

2. Is the Tribunal satisfied that it is not necessary for the health or safety of the patient or for the protection of other persons that the patient should receive such treatment?   Yes/No

If the answers to both questions 1 and 2 are 'No', does the Tribunal consider that this is a case in which it is appropriate to discharge the patient under its discretionary power?

Part VII

Medico-legal
Aspects of
Psychiatry

Professional bodies

British Medical Association
Tavistock Square
London WC1H 9JP
Tel: (0171) 3874499
(Head Office)

Royal College of Psychiatrists
17 Belgrave Square
London SW1X 8PG
Tel: (0171) 2352351
Fax: (0171) 2451231

Enquiries about the code of practice

Department of Health
Alexander Fleming House
Elephant and Castle
London SE1 6BY
Tel: (0171) 2105983

Welsh Office
Cathays Park
Cardiff CF1 3NQ
Tel: (01222) 825111

Adverse drug reactions
These should be reported to:

CSM
Freepost
London SW8 5BR
(0171) 6273291

General addresses

Age Concern Greater London
54 Knatchbull Road
London SE5 9QU
Tel: (0171) 2746723

Age Concern Wales
1 Cathedral Road
Cardiff CF1 9SD
Tel: (01222) 371566

Age Concern Scotland
54A Fountain Bridge
Edinburgh EH3 9PT
Tel: (0131) 2285656

Age Concern Northern Ireland
3 Lower Crescent
Belfast BT7 1NR
Tel: (01232) 245729

Alzheimer's Disease Society
2nd Floor, Gordon House
10 Greencoat Place
London SW1P 1PH
Tel: (0171) 3060606

Association of Continence Advisers
Disabled Living Foundation
380–4 Harrow Road
London W9 2HU
Tel: (0171) 2663704

British Association of Occupational Therapists
6 Marshalsea Road
London SE1 1HL
Tel: (0171) 3576480

British Geriatrics Society (BGS)
1 St Andrews Place
Regents Park

London NW1 4LB
Tel: (0171) 9354004

British Red Cross
9 Grosvenor Crescent
London SW1X 7EJ
Tel: (0171) 2355454

**Campaign for Single
    Homeless People
    (CHAR)**
5–15 Cromer Street
London WC1
Tel: (0171) 8332071

**Centre for Policy on
    Ageing (CPA)**
25–31 Ironmonger Row
London EC1V 3QP
Tel: (0171) 2531787

**Chartered Society of
    Physiotherapy**
14 Bedford Row
London WC1R 4ED
Tel: (0171) 2421941

**Community Service
    Volunteers**
237 Pentonville Road
Kings Cross
London N1 9NG
Tel: (0171) 2786001

**Counsel and Care for
    the Elderly**
Twyman House
16 Bonny Street
NW1 9PG
Tel: (0171) 4851550

Court of Protection
Stewart House
24 Kingsway

London WC2B 6HD
Tel: (0171) 2697000

Disability Alliance
Universal House
Wentworth Street
London E1 7SA
Tel: (0171) 2478776

**Disabled Living
    Foundation**
380–4 Harrow Road
London W9 2HU
Tel: (0171) 2896111

**Health Education
    Authority**
Hamilton House
Mabledon Place
London WC1
Tel: (0171) 3879528

Help the Aged
St James' Walk
London EC1R 0BE
Tel: (0171) 2530253

Jewish Care
221 Golders Green
    Road
London NW11 9DZ
Tel: (0181) 4583282

King's Fund Centre
126 Albert Street
London NW1 7NF
Tel: (0171) 2676111

**MIND – National
    Association for
    Mental Health**
22 Harley Street
London W1N 2ED
Tel: (0171) 6370741

National Association of Citizens Advice Bureaux
115 Pentonville Road
London N1 9LZ
Tel: (0171) 8332181

National Council for Voluntary Organizations (NCVO)
26 Bedford Square
London WC1B 3HU
Tel: (0171) 6364066

Parkinson's Disease Society
36 Portland Place
London W1N 3DG
Tel: (0171) 3833513

Royal Association for Disability and Rehabilitation (RADAR)
25 Mortimer Street
London W1N 8AB
Tel: (0171) 6375400

Royal National Institute for the Blind
224 Great Portland Street
London W1N 4XX
Tel: (0171) 3881266

Shape
1 Thorpe Close
London W10 5XL
Tel: (0181) 9609245

St John Ambulance
1 Grosvenor Crescent
London SW1X 7EE
Tel: (0171) 2355231

Terrence Higgins Trust
52/54 Gray's Inn Road
London WC1X 8JU
Tel: (0171) 2421010
(12 noon-7 p.m. daily)

Principal government offices

Advisory, Conciliation and Arbitration Services
Clifton House
83–117 Euston Road
London NW1 2RB
Tel: (0171) 3960002

Agricultural Ministry of Fisheries & Foods
Place Whitehall
East Block Whitehall
London SW1A 2HH
Tel: (0171) 2386000

Bank of England
Threadneedle Street
London EC2R 8AH
Tel: (0171) 6014444

Central Office of Information
Hercules Road
London SE1 7DU
Tel: (0171) 9282345

Central Office of the Industrial Tribunals
100 Southgate Street
Bury St Edmunds
Suffolk IP33 2AO
Tel: (01284) 762300

Central Statistical Office
Government Building
Cardiff Road, Newport
Gwent NP9 1XG
Tel: (01633) 812973

Commission for Local Administration in England
21 Queen Anne's Gate
London SW1H 9BU
Tel: (0171) 9153210

Commission for Racial Equality
Elliot House
10–12 Allington Street
London SW1E 5EH
Tel: (0171) 8287022

Commonwealth Development Corporation
One Bessborough Gardens
London SW1V 2JQ
Tel: (0171) 8284488

Companies Registration Office
Companies House
Crown Way
Cardiff CF4 3U7
Tel: (01222) 380801

Consumer Affairs Division
1 Victoria Street
London SW1H 0ET
Tel: (0171) 2155000

Crown Prosecution Service
50 Ludgate Hill
London EC4M 7EX
Tel: (0171) 2733000

Customs and Excise, HM
New Kings Beam House
22 Upper Ground
London SE1 9PJ
Tel: (0171) 6201313

Defence, Ministry of
Main Building
Whitehall
London SW1A 2HB
Tel: (0171) 2189000

Education & Employment, Department for
Sanctuary Buildings
Great Smith Street
Westminster SW1P 3BT
Tel: (0171) 9255000

Employment, Department of
Caxton House
Lothill Street
London SW1H 9NF
Tel: (0171) 2733000

Environment, Department of the
2 Marsham Street
London SW1P 3EB
Tel: (0171) 2760900

Equal Opportunities Commission
Overseas House
Quay Street
Manchester M3 3HN
Tel: (0161) 8339244

Export Credits Guarantee Department
2 Exchange Tower
Harbour Exchange
Square
London E14 9GS
Tel: (0171) 5127000

Export Market Information Centre
Kingsgate House
66–74 Victoria Street
London SW1E 6RB
Tel: (0171) 2155444

Foreign & Commonwealth Office
King Charles Street
London SW1A 2AH
Tel: (0171) 2703000

Health & Safety Executive (General Enquiries)
Broad Lane
Sheffield S3 7HQ
Tel: (01142) 892000

Health, Department of
Richmond House
79 Whitehall
London SW1A 2NS
Tel: (0171) 2104850

Home Office
50 Queen Anne's Gate
London SW1H 9AT
Tel: (0171) 2733000

Inland Revenue, Board of
Somerset House
The Strand
London WC2R 1LB
Tel: (0171) 4386420

London Tax Enquiry Centre
Charles House
375 Kensington High
Street
London W14 8RO
Tel: (0171) 6059800

Inland Revenue Central Purchasing Unit & Board of Investigation
Lynwood Road
Thames Ditton
Surrey KT7 0DP
Tel: (0181) 3984242

Special Commissioners of Income Tax
15–19 Bedford
Avenue
London WC1B 3AS
Tel: (0171) 6314242

Meteorological Office
London Road
Bracknell
Berkshire RG12 2SZ
Tel: (01344) 420242

Monopolies & Mergers Commission
New Court
48 Carey Street
London WC2A 2JT
Tel: (0171) 8241467

National Audit Office
157–197 Buckingham Palace Road
London SW1W 9SP
Tel: (0171) 7987000

National Consumer Council
20 Grosvenor Gardens
London SW1W 0DH
Tel: (0171) 7303469

Northern Ireland Office
Stormont Castle
Stormont Estate
Belfast BT4 3ST
Tel: (01232) 520700

Office of Fair Trading
Field House
15–25 Bream's Buildings
London EC4A 1PR
Tel: (0171) 2422858

Office of Population Censuses & Surveys/ General Register Office
St Catherine's House
10 Kingsway
London WC2B 6JP
Tel: (0171) 2420262

Overseas Development Administration
94 Victoria Street
London SW1E 5JL
Tel: (0171) 9177000

Patent Office
Cardiff Road, Newport
Gwent NP9 1XG
Tel: (01633) 814000

Public Record Office
Ruskin Avenue
Kew, Richmond Surrey
TW9 4DU
Tel: (0181) 8763444

Social Security, Department of
Richmond House
79 Whitehall
London SW1A 2NS
Tel: (0171) 2105983

Stationery Office, HM
Publications Centre
PO Box 276
London SW8 5DT
Tel: (0171) 8730011

Scottish Office
St Andrews House
Regent Road
Edinburgh EH1 3DG
Tel: (0131) 5568400

Trade & Industry, Department of
Enquiry Unit
1 Victoria Street
London SW1H 0ET
Tel: (0171) 2155000

Telecommunications & Post

151 Buckingham Palace Road
London SW1W 9SS
Tel: (0171) 2155000

Transport, Department of

Great Minster House
76 Marsham Street
London SW1P 4DR
Tel: (0171) 271500
Public Enquiries:
(0171) 2714800

Treasury, HM

Parliament Street
London SW1P 3AG
Tel: (0171) 2703000

Welsh Office

Crown Building
Cathays Park
Cardiff CF1 3NQ
Tel: (01222) 825111

Regional tribunal offices
Mental Health Review Tribunals
Hepburn House
Marsham Street
London SW1P 4HW
Tel: (0171) 211325
(0171) 211356

Mental Health Review Tribunals
3rd floor
Cressington House
249 St Mary's Road
Garston

Liverpool L19 0NF
Tel: (0151) 494 0095

Mental Health Review Tribunals
Spur A, Block 5
Government Buildings
Chalfont Drive
Western Boulevard
Nottingham NG8 3RZ
Tel: (0115) 94222/3

Mental Health Review Tribunals
2nd Floor
New Crown Buildings
Cathays Park
Cardiff CF1 3NQ
Tel: (01222) 825798

Department of Health and Social Security
Mental Health Division
Alexander Fleming House
Elephant & Castle
London SE1 6BY
Tel: (0171) 407 5522

Mental Health Act Commission (regional offices)
London Office
Floors 1 and 2
Hepburn House
Marsham Street
London SW1P 4HW
Tel: (0171) 211 8061
(0171) 211 4337

Liverpool Office
Cressington House
249 St Mary's Road

Garston
Liverpool L19 0NF
Tel: (0151) 427 2061
(0151) 427 6213

Nottingham Office
Spur A, Block 5
Government Buildings
Chalfont Drive
Western Boulevard
Nottingham NG8 3R2
Tel: (0115) 9293409
(0115) 9293198

Court of Protection
Chief Clerk
Court of Protection
Staffordshire House
25 Store Street
London WC1E 7BP
Tel: (0171) 636 6877

C3 Division, Home Office
C3 Division
Home Office
50 Queen Anne's Gate
London SW1H 9AT
Tel: (0171) 213 7355

*Law Society – Legal Aid
Area Centres (England
and Wales)*
No. 1 London South
The Law Society
No 1 Legal Aid Area
Area Headquarters
29/37 Red Lion Street
London WC1R 4PP
Tel: (0171) 4056991

No. 2 South-Eastern
The Law Society
No. 2 Legal Aid Area

Area Headquarters
9–12 Middle Street
Brighton BN1 1AS
Tel: (01273) 27003

No. 3 Southern
The Law Society
No. 3 Legal Aid Area
Area Headquarters
Crown House
10 Crown Street
Reading RG1 2SJ
Tel: (01734) 589696

No. 4 South-Western
The Law Society
No. 4 Legal Aid Area
Area Headquarters
Whitefriars (Block 'C')
Lewis Mead
Bristol BS1 2LR
Tel: (01272) 214801

No. 5 South Wales
The Law Society
No. 5 Legal Aid Area
Area Headquarters
Marland House
Central Square
Cardiff CF1 1PE
Tel: (01222) 388971/7

No. 6 West-Midland
The Law Society
No. 6 Legal Aid Area
Area Headquarters
Podium
Centre City House
5 Hill Street
Birmingham B5 4UD
Tel: (0121) 632 6541

No. 7 North-Western
The Law Society
No. 7 Legal Aid Area
Area Headquarters
Pall Mall Court
67 King Street
Manchester M60 9AX
Tel: (0161) 832 7112

No. 8 Northern
The Law Society
No. 8 Legal Aid Area
Area Headquarters
18 Newgate Shopping
  Centre
Newcastle Upon Tyne
NE1 5RU
Tel: (01632) 23461/4

No. 9 North-Eastern
The Law Society
No. 9 Legal Aid Area
Area Headquarters
City House
New Station Street
Leeds LS1 4JS
Tel: (01532) 442851/6

No. 10 East-Midland
The Law Society
No. 10 Legal Aid Area
Area Headquarters
5 Friar Lane
Nottingham NG1 6BW
Tel: (0115) 942341/4

No. 11 Eastern
The Law Society
No. 11 Legal Aid Area
Area Headquarters
Kett House
Station Road

Cambridge CB1 2JT
Tel: (01223) 66511/7

No. 12 Chester and
  District
The Law Society
No. 12 Legal Aid Area
Area Headquarters
North West House
City Road
Chester CH1 2AL
Tel: (01244) 23591

No. 13 London-East
The Law Society
No. 13 Legal Aid Area
Area Headquarters
29/37 Red Lion Street
London WC1R 4PP
Tel: (0171) 405 6991

No. 14 London-West
The Law Society
No 14 Legal Aid Area
Area Headquarters
29/37 Red Lion Street
London WC1R 4PP
Tel: (0171) 405 6991

No. 15 Merseyside
The Law Society
No. 15 Legal Aid Area
Area Headquarters
Moor House
James Street
Liverpool L2 7SA
Tel: (0151) 236 8371

Manufacturers
Abbott
Abbott Laboratories
  Ltd
Abbott House

Norden Road
Maidenhead
Berks SL6 4XE
(01628) 773355

A&H
Allen & Hanburys Ltd,
see Glaxo Wellcome

Alcon
Alcon Laboratories
(UK) Ltd
Pentagon Park
Boundary Way
Hemel Hempstead
Herts HP2 7UD
(01442) 341234

Alembic Products
Alembic Products Ltd
River Lane
Saltney
Chester
Cheshire CH4 8RQ
(01244) 680147

ALK
ALK (UK)
8 Bennet Road
Reading
Berks RG2 0QX
(01734) 313200

Allerayde
Allerayde
3 Sanigar Court
Whittle Close
Newark
Notts NG24 2BW
(01636) 613444

Allergan
Allergan Ltd

Coronation Road
High Wycombe
Bucks HP12 3SH
(01494) 444722

Alpha
Alpha Therapeutic UK
Ltd
Howlett Way
Fison Way Industrial
Estate
Thetford
Norfolk IP24 1HZ
(01842) 764260

AlphaMed
AlphaMed Ltd
Bensham House
340 Bensham Lane
Thornton Heath
Surrey CR7 7EQ
0181–684 0470

Amersham
Amersham
International plc
Amersham Place
Little Chalfont
Bucks HP7 9NA,
(01494) 544000

Amgen
Amgen Ltd
240 Cambridge Science
Park
Milton Road
Cambridge CB4 4WD
(01223) 420305

Anpharm
Anpharm Ltd
82 Waterloo Road

Hillside
Southport PR8 4QW.

Antigen
Antigen Pharma-
ceuticals (UK)
Trafalgar House
Union Street
Southport
Merseyside PR9 0QS
(01704) 545608

APS
Approved Prescription
Services Ltd
Brampton Road
Hampden Park
Eastbourne
East Sussex BN22 9AG
(01323) 501111

Armour
Armour Pharma-
ceutical Co. Ltd
RPR House
52 St. Leonards Road
Eastbourne
East Sussex BN21 3YG
(01323) 410200

Ashbourne
Ashbourne
Pharmaceuticals Ltd
Victors Barns
Hill Farm
Brixworth
Northampton
NN6 9DQ
(01604) 882190

ASTA Medica
ASTA Medica Ltd
168 Cowley Road

Cambridge CB4 4DL
(01223) 423434

Astra
Astra Pharmaceuticals
Ltd
Home Park Estate
Kings Langley
Herts WD4 8DH
(01923) 266191

Astra Tech
Astra Tech Ltd
Stroudwater Business
Park
Brunel Way
Stonehouse
Glos GL10 3SW
(01453) 791763

Aurum
Aurum
Pharmaceuticals Ltd
48–50 High Street
Billingshurst
West Sussex RH14 9NY
(01403) 786781

Bailey, Robert
Robert Bailey & Son
plc
Dysart Street
Great Moor
Stockport
Cheshire SK2 7PF
0161–483 1133

Baker Norton
Division of Norton
Healthcare, *see*
Norton

Bard
Bard Ltd

Forest House
Brighton Road
Crawley
West Sussex RH11 9BP
(01293) 527888

Baxter
Baxter Healthcare Ltd
Caxton Way
Thetford
Norfolk IP24 3SE
(01842) 767000

Bayer
Bayer plc
Pharmaceutical
  Business Group
Bayer House
Strawberry Hill
Newbury
Berks RG13 1JA
(01635) 39000

Bayer Diagnostics
Bayer Diagnostics
Evans House
Hamilton Close
Houndmills
Basingstoke
Hants RG21 2YE
(01256) 29181

Baypharm
see Bayer

BCM Specials
Boots Contract
  Manufacturing
1 Thane Road West
Nottingham NG2 3AA
0500 925935

Becton Dickinson
Becton Dickinson UK
  Ltd
Between Towns Road
Cowley
Oxford
Oxon OX4 3LY
(01865) 748844

Beecham
Beecham Research, *see*
  SmithKline Beecham

Beecham Products
see SmithKline
  Beecham Healthcare

Beiersdorf
Beiersdorf UK Ltd
Yeomans Drive
Blakelands
Milton Keynes
Bucks MK14 5LS
(01908) 211444

Bell and Croyden
John Bell and Croyden
54 Wigmore Street
London W1H 0AU
0171–935 5555

Bencard
see SmithKline
  Beecham

Bengué
Bengué & Co Ltd, *see*
  Syntex

Berk
Berk Pharmaceuticals,
  see APS

Beta
Beta Medical Products
  Ltd

Valley Lodge
Bakewell Road
Matlock
Derbyshire DE4 3BN
(01629) 582198

BHR

BHR Pharmaceuticals
  Ltd
41 Centenary Business
  Centre
Hammond Close
Attleborough Fields
Nuneaton
Warwickshire CV11 6RY
(01203) 353742

Bio Diagnostics

Bio Diagnostics Ltd
Upton Industrial Estate
Rectory Road
Upton-upon-Severn
Worcs WR8 0XL
(01684) 592262

Biocare

Biocare International
  Inc.
Belvoir House
Chapel Street
Haconby
Lincs PE10 0UP
(01778) 570441

Bioglan

Bioglan Laboratories
  Ltd
5 Hunting Gate
Hitchin
Herts SG4 0TJ
(01462) 438444

Bio-Medical

Bio-Medical Services
BMS Laboratories Ltd
River View Road
Beverley
North Humberside
HU17 0LD
(01482) 860228

Biorex

Biorex Laboratories
  Ltd
2 Crossfield Chambers
Gladbeck Way
Enfield
Middx EN2 7HT
0181–366 9301

Blake

Thomas Blake & Co
The Byre House
Fearby
Nr. Masham
North Yorkshire
HG4 4NF
(01765) 689042

BM Diagnostics

Boehringer Mannheim
(Diagnostics &
  Biochemicals)Ltd
Bell Lane
Lewes
East Sussex BN7 1LG
(01273) 480444

BOC

BOC Gases
Priestly Rd
Worsley
Manchester M28 2UT
0800 111333

Body's Surgical
Body's Surgical
  Company
Unit 14
East Hanningfield
  Industrial Estate
Old Church Road
East Hanningfield
Chelmsford
Essex CM3 8BG
(01245) 400413

Boehringer Ingelheim
Boehringer Ingelheim
  Ltd
Ellesfield Avenue
Bracknell
Berks RG12 4YS
(01344) 424600

Boehringer Mannheim
Boehringer Mannheim
  UK (Pharma-
  ceuticals) Ltd
Simpson Parkway
Kirkton Campus
Livingston
West Lothian
EH54 7BH
(01506) 412512

Boots
The Boots Co plc
1 Thane Road West
Nottingham NG2 3AA
(0115) 959 5168

BPL
Bio Products
  Laboratory
Dagger Lane
Elstree

Herts WD6 3BX
0181–905 1818

Braun
B. Braun (Medical) Ltd
Braun House
13–14 Farmbrough
  Close
Aylesbury
Vale Industrial Park
Aylesbury
Bucks HP20 1DQ
(01296) 393900

Bristol-Myers
Bristol-Myers Squibb
Pharmaceuticals Ltd
141–149 Staines Road
Hounslow
Middx TW3 3JA
0181–572 7422

Britannia
Britannia
  Pharmaceuticals Ltd
41–51 Brighton Road
Redhill
Surrey RH1 6YS
(01737) 773741

David Bull
David Bull Laboratories
Spartan Close
Tachbrook Park
Warwick CV34 6RS
(01926) 820820

Bullen
C. S. Bullen Ltd
3–7 Moss Street
Liverpool L6 1EY
0151–207 6995

Bullen & Smears
Bullen & Smears Ltd,
  see Bullen

Burgess
Edwin Burgess Ltd, *see*
  Leo

Cambridge
Cambridge
  Laboratories
Richmond House
Old Brewery Court
Sandyford Road
Newcastle upon Tyne
NE2 1XG
0191–261 5950

Camp
Camp Ltd
30–32 Sovereign Road
Kings Norton Business
  Centre
Birmingham B30 3HN
0121–451 3016

Cantassium
The Cantassium
  Company
Larkhall Laboratories
225 Putney Bridge
  Road
London SW15 2PY
0181–874 1130

Centra
Centra Healthcare
Enterprise House
Station Road
Loudwater
High Wycombe
Bucks HP10 9UF
(01494) 450778

Chancellor
Chancellor Group Ltd,
  see Consolidated

Chauvin
Chauvin
  Pharmaceuticals Ltd
Ashton Road
Harold Hill
Romford
Essex RM3 8SL
(01708) 383838

J. Chawner
J. Chawner Surgical
  Belts Ltd
Unit 1B Mayfields
Southcrest
Redditch B98 7DU
(01527) 404353

Chefaro
Chefaro Proprietaries
  Ltd, *see* Organon
(01223) 420956

Chiron
Chiron UK Ltd
Salamander Quay West
Park Lane
Harefield
Middx UB9 6NY
(01895) 824087

Chugai
Chugai Pharma UK Ltd
Mulliner House
Flanders Road
Turnham Green
London W4 1NN
0181–742 0777

Ciba
Ciba Pharmaceuticals

Wimblehurst Road
Horsham
West Sussex RH12 4AB
(01403) 272827

CIBA Vision
CIBA Vision
Ophthalmics
Flanders Road
Hedge End
Southampton
SO30 2LG
(01489) 785399

Cilag
see Janssen-Cilag

Clement Clarke
Clement Clarke
International Ltd
Airmed House
Edinburgh Way
Harlow
Essex CM20 2ED
(01279) 414969

CliniFlex
CliniFlex Ltd, *see*
CliniMed

CliniMed
CliniMed Ltd
Cavell House
Knaves Beech Way
Loudwater
High Wycombe
Bucks HP10 9QY
(01628) 850100

Clintec
Clintec Nutrition Ltd
Shaftesbury Court
18 Chalvey Park

Slough
Berks SL1 2ER
(01753) 550800

Colgate-Palmolive
Colgate-Palmolive Ltd
Guildford Business
Park
Middleton Road
Guildford
Surrey GU2 5LZ
(01483) 302222

Coloplast
Coloplast Ltd
Peterborough Business
Park
Peterborough PE2 0FX
(01733) 239898

Consolidated
Consolidated
Chemicals Ltd
Abbey Road
The Industrial Estate
Wrexham
Clywd LL13 9PW
(01978) 661351

ConvaTec
ConvaTec Ltd
Harrington House
Milton Road
Ickenham
Uxbridge
Middx UB10 8PU
(01895) 678888

Co-Pharma
Co-Pharma Ltd
Talbot House
Church Street
Rickmansworth

Herts WD3 1DE
(01923) 710934

Cover Care
Cover Care
5 Ancaster Gardens
Wollaton Park
Nottingham NG8 1FR
(0115) 928 7883

Cow & Gate
Cow & Gate Nutricia
    Ltd
Newmarket Avenue
White Horse Business
    Park
Trowbridge
Wilts BA14 0XQ
(01225) 768381

Cox
A. H. Cox & Co Ltd
Whiddon Valley
Barnstaple
Devon EX32 8NS
(01271) 311257

CP
CP Pharmaceuticals
    Ltd
Ash Road North
Wrexham Industrial
    Estate
Wrexham
Clwyd LL13 9UP
(01978) 661261

Crawford
Crawford
    Pharmaceuticals
71a High Street
Stony Stratford
Milton Keynes

MK11 1BA
(01908) 262346

Credenhill
Credenhill Ltd
10 Cossall Industrial
    Estate
Ilkeston
Derbys DE7 5UG
(0115) 932 0144

Crookes
Crookes Healthcare
    Ltd
PO Box 57
Central Park
Lenton Lane
Nottingham NG7 2LJ
(0115) 953 9922

Cupal
Cupal Ltd, *See* Seton

Cupharma
Cupharma Ltd
Winkton House
Wynnswick Road
Seer Green
Beaconsfield
Bucks HP9 2XW
(01494) 677055

Cussons
Cussons (UK) Ltd
Kersal Vale
Manchester M7 0GL
0161–792 6111

Cutter
see Bayer

Cuxson
Cuxson, Gerrard & Co
    Ltd

Oldbury
Warley
West Midlands B69 4BF
0121–544 7117

Daniels
see Martindale

Dansac
Dansac Ltd
Victory House
Vision Park
Histon
Cambridge CB4 4ZR
(01223) 235100

Davis & Geck
see Lederle

DDC
DDC (London) Ltd
6 Clifton Gardens
London W9 1DT
0171–266 0056

DDD
DDD Ltd
94 Rickmansworth Rd
Watford
Herts WD1 7JJ
(01923) 229251

DDSA
DDSA Pharmaceuticals
    Ltd
310 Old Brompton
    Road
London SW5 9JQ
0171–373 7884

De Vilbiss
De Vilbiss Health Care
    UK Ltd
Airlinks

Spitfire Way
Heston
Middx TW5 9NR
0181–756 1133

De Witt
E. C. De Witt & Co Ltd
Tudor Road
Manor Park
Runcorn
Cheshire WA7 1SZ
(01928) 579029

Delandale
Delandale Laboratories
    Ltd, *see* Lorex

Dental Health
Dental Health Products
    Ltd
Pearl Assurance House
Mill Street
Maidstone
Kent ME15 6XH
(01622) 762269

DePuy
DePuy Healthcare
Millshaw House
Manor Mill Lane
Leeds LS11 8LQ
(0113) 270 6000

Dermal
Dermal Laboratories
    Ltd
Tatmore Place
Gosmore
Hitchin
Herts SG4 7QR
(01462) 458866

Dermalex
see Sanofi Winthrop

DF
Duncan, Flockhart &
  Co Ltd
Division of Glaxo
  Wellcome Ltd
see Glaxo Wellcome

Dista
Dista Products Ltd, *see*
  Lilly.

Dominion
Dominion Pharma Ltd
Dominion House
Lion Lane
Haslemere
Surrey GU27 1JL
(01428) 661078

Downs
see Simcare

Drew
John Drew (London)
  Ltd
433 Uxbridge Road
Ealing
London W5 3NT
0181–992 0381

Du Pont
Du Pont
  Pharmaceuticals Ltd
Avenue One
Letchworth
Garden City
Herts SG6 2HU
(01462) 482648

Dumex
Dumex Ltd
Tring Business Centre
Upper Icknield Way

Tring
Herts HP23 4JX
(01442) 890090

Durbin
B & S Durbin Ltd
240 Northolt Road
South Harrow
Middx HA2 8DU
0181–422 1303

Dylade
see Fresenius

Eastern
Eastern
  Pharmaceuticals Ltd
Coomb House
7 St Johns Road
Isleworth
Middx TW7 6NA
0181–569 8174

Elan
Elan Pharma Ltd, *see*
  P-D.

Elida Gibbs
Elida Gibbs Ltd
Coal Road
Seacroft
Leeds LS14 2AR
(0113) 273 7473

Ellis
Ellis, Son & Paramore
  Ltd, *see* Camp

EMS
EMS Medical Ltd
Unit 3, Stroud
  Industrial Estate
Stonedale Road
Oldends Lane

Stonehouse
Glos GL10 2DG
(01453) 791791

Ethical Generics Ltd
Ethical Generics Ltd
West Point
46–48 West Street
Newbury
Berkshire RG14 1BD
(01635) 568406

EuroCare
EuroCare (UK) Ltd
55 Wimpole Street
London W1M 7DF
0171–935 8560

Euroderma
Euroderma Ltd
The Old Coach House
34 Elm Road
Chessington
Surrey KT9 1AW
0181–974 2266

Evans
Evans Medical Ltd
Evans House
Regent Park
Kingston Road
Leatherhead
Surrey KT22 7PQ
(01372) 364000

Everfresh
Everfresh Natural
  Foods
Gatehouse Close
Aylesbury
Bucks HP19 3DE
(01296) 25333

Farillon
Farillon Ltd
Ashton Road
Harold Hill
Romford
Essex RM3 8UE
(01708) 379000

Farley
Farley Health Products
Mint Bridge Road
Kendal
Cumbria LA9 6NL
(01539) 723815

Ferraris
Ferraris Development
  & Engineering Co
  Ltd
26 Lea Valley Trading
  Estate
Angel Road
Edmonton
London N18 3JD
0181–807 3636

Ferring
Ferring
  Pharmaceuticals Ltd
Greville House
Hatton Road
Feltham
Middx TW14 9PX
0181–893 1543

Fisons
Fisons plc
Pharmaceutical
  Division
Coleorton Hall
Ashby Road
Coleorton

Coalville
Leics LE67 8GP
(01509) 634000

Flynn
Flynn Pharma Ltd
7 Serlby Court
Addison Road
London W14 8EE
(01438) 820152

Forley
Forley Ltd
54 Hillbury Avenue
Harrow
Middx HA3 8EW
0181–665 9169

Fournier
Fournier
    Pharmaceuticals Ltd
19–20 Progress
    Business Centre
White Parkway
Slough SL1 6DQ
(01628) 660552

Fox
C. H. Fox Ltd
22 Tavistock Street
London WC2E 7PY
0171–240 3111

FP
Family Planning Sales
    Ltd
28 Kelburne Road
Cowley
Oxford OX4 3SZ
(01865) 772486

Fresenius
Fresenius Ltd

6–8 Christleton Court
Stuart Road
Manor Park
Runcorn
Cheshire WA7 1ST
(01928) 579444

Fry
Fry Surgical
    International Ltd
Unit 17
Goldsworth Park
    Trading Estate
Woking
Surrey GU21 3BA
(01483) 721404

Fujisawa
Fujisawa Ltd
C P House, 8th Floor
97–107 Uxbridge Road
London W5 5TL
0181–840 9520

Gainor Medical
Gainor Medical Europe
Milton Keynes
    Distribution Centre
Bradbourne Drive
Tilbrook
Milton Keynes
MK7 8BN
(01908) 365361

Galderma
Galderma (UK) Ltd
Leywood House
Woodside Road
Amersham
Bucks HP6 6AA
(01494) 432606

Galen
Galen Ltd
Seagoe Industrial
  Estate
Craigavon
Northern Ireland
BT63 5UA
(01762) 334974

Garnier
Laboratoires Garnier
Golden Ltd
PO Box 5
Pontyclun
Glam CF7 8XW
(01443) 237456

Geigy
Geigy Pharmaceuticals,
  see Ciba.

Geistlich
Geistlich Sons Ltd
Newton Bank
Long Lane
Chester CH2 2PF
(01244) 347534

General Dietary
General Dietary Ltd
PO Box 38
Kingston upon Thames
Surrey KT2 7YP
0181-336 2323

Generics
Generics (UK) Ltd
12 Station Close
Potters Bar
Herts EN6 1TL
(01707) 644556

Gensia
Gensia Europe Ltd

1 Bracknell Beeches
Bracknell
Berks RG12 7BW
(01334) 308803

GF Supplies
see Nutricia

Glaxo
see Glaxo Wellcome

GlaxoWellcome
GlaxoWellcome Ltd
Stockley Park West
Uxbridge
Middx UB11 1BT
0181-990 9444

Glenwood
Glenwood Laboratories
  Ltd
Jenkins Dale
Chatham
Kent ME4 5RD
(01634) 830535

Gluten Free Foods Ltd
Gluten Free Foods Ltd
PO Box 178
Stanmore
Middx HA7 4XN
0181-954 7348

Goldshield
Goldshield
  Pharmaceuticals Ltd
NLA Tower
12–16 Addiscombe
  Road
Croydon
Surrey CR9 6BP
0181-649 8500

Henleys
Henleys Medical
   Supplies Ltd
Brownfields
Welwyn Garden City
Herts AL7 1AN
(01707) 333164

Hillcross
Hillcross
   Pharmaceuticals
Talbot Street
Briercliffe
Burnley BB10 2JY
(01282) 830042

Hoechst
see Hoechst Roussel

Hoechst Roussel
Hoechst Roussel Ltd
Broadwater Park
Denham
Uxbridge
Middx UB9 5HP
(01895) 834343

Hollister
Hollister Ltd
Rectory Court
42 Broad Street
Wokingham
Berks RG11 1AB
(01734) 775545

**Hospital Management
   & Supplies**
Hospital Management
   and Supplies Ltd
Salthouse Road
Brackmills
Northampton

NN4 7UF
(01604) 704600

Houghs
Houghs Healthcare Ltd
18–22 Chapel Street
Manchester M19 3PT
0161–224 3271

Hutchings
Hutchings Healthcare
   Ltd
Rede House
New Barn Lane
Henfield
West Sussex BN5 9SJ
(01273) 495033

Hypoguard
Hypoguard Ltd
Dock Lane
Melton
Woodbridge
Suffolk IP12 1PE
(01394) 387333

IATRO
IATRO Medical
   Systems
35 Quaggy Walk
Blackheath
London SE3 9EJ
0181–297 9081

ICN
ICN Pharmaceuticals
   Inc
Eagle House
Peregrine Business
   Park
Gomm Road
High Wycombe

Bucks HP13 7DL
(01494) 444555

IDIS
IDIS Ltd
6/7 Canbury Business
    Park
Elm Crescent
Kingston upon Thames
Surrey KT2 6BR
0181–549 1355

Immuno
Immuno Ltd
Arctic House
Rye Lane
Dunton Green
Nr Sevenoaks
Kent TN14 5HB
(01732) 458101

Impharm
Impharm Nationwide
    Ltd
PWS Building
Nelson Street
Bolton BL3 2JW
(01204) 371155

IMS
International
    Medication Systems
    (UK) Ltd
Foster Avenue
Woodside Park Estate
Dunstable
Beds LU5 5TA
(01582) 475005

Incare
Incare Medical
    Products, *see*
    Hollister.

Innovex
Innovex Medical, *see*
    Novex.

Intercare
Intercare Products Ltd
7 The Business Centre
Molly Millars Lane
Wokingham
Berks RG41 2QZ
(01734) 790345

Invicta
see Pfizer

ISIS
ISIS Products Ltd
Gough Lane
Bamber Bridge
Preston
Lancs PR5 6AQ
(01772) 628311

J&J
Johnson & Johnson Ltd
Foundation Park
Roxborough Way
Maidenhead
Berkshire SL6 3UG
(01628) 822222

J&J Medical
Johnson & Johnson
    Medical
Coronation Road
Ascot
Berks SL5 9EY
(01344) 872626

Jacobs
The Jacobs Bakery Ltd
Suttons Business Park
Earley

Reading
Berks RG6 1AZ
(01734) 492000

Janssen
see Janssen-Cilag

Janssen-Cilag
Janssen-Cilag Ltd
PO Box 79
Saunderton
High Wycombe
Bucks HP14 4HJ
(01494) 567567

JLB
JLB Textiles Ltd
Unit 2B, St Columb
    Industrial Estate
St Columb Major
Cornwall TR9 6SF
(01637) 880065

K & K-Greeff
K & K-Greeff Ltd
Suffolk House
George Street
Croydon CR9 3QL
0181–686 0544

K/L
K/L Pharmaceuticals
    Ltd
25 Macadam Place
South Newmoor
    Industrial Estate
Irvine KA11 4HP
(01294) 215951

Kendall
The Kendall Co (UK)
    Ltd
2 Elmwood, Chineham
    Business Park

Crockford Lane
Basingstoke
Hants RG24 0WG
(01256) 708880

Kendall-Lastonet
see Kendall

Kent
Kent Pharmaceuticals
    Ltd
Wotton Road
Ashford
Kent TN23 6LL
(01233) 641802

Kestrel
Kestrel Healthcare Ltd
21a Hyde Street
Winchester
Hants SO23 7DR
(01962) 866449

Kimal
Kimal Scientific
    Products Ltd
Arundel Road
Uxbridge
Middx UB8 2SA
(01895) 270951

Knoll
Knoll Ltd
9 Castle Quay
Castle Boulevard
Nottingham NG7 1FW
(0115) 912 5000

Kyowa Hakko
Kyowa Hakko UK Ltd
CP House
97–107 Uxbridge Road
Ealing

London W5 5TL
0181–840 4600

LAB
Laboratories for
    Applied Biology Ltd
91 Amhurst Park
London N16 5DR.
0181–800 2252

Laerdal
Laerdal Medical Ltd
Laerdal House
Goodmead Road
Orpington
Kent BR6 0HX
(01689) 876634

Lagap
Lagap Pharmaceuticals
    Ltd
37 Woolmer Way
Bordon
Hants GU35 9QE
(01420) 478301

Lamberts
Lamberts (Dalston) Ltd
Dalston House
Hastings Street
Luton
Beds LU1 5BW
(01582) 400711

Lederle
Lederle Laboratories,
    see Wyeth

Lennon
see Trinity

Leo
Leo Laboratories Ltd
Longwick Road

Princes Risborough
Aylesbury
Bucks HP27 9RR
(01844) 347333

LifeScan
LifeScan
Enterprise House
Station Road
Loudwater
High Wycombe
Bucks HP10 9UF
(01494) 442211

Lilly
Eli Lilly & Co Ltd
Dextra Court
Chapel Hill
Basingstoke
Hants RG21 5SY
(01256) 315000

Link
Link Pharmaceuticals
    Ltd
51 Bishopric
Horsham
West Sussex RH12 1QJ
(01403) 272451

Lipha
Lipha Pharmaceuticals
    Ltd, *see* Merck

Liposome Company
The Liposome Co Ltd
3 Shortlands
Hammersmith
    International Centre
London W6 8EH
0181–324 0058

Lorex
Lorex Synthélabo Ltd

Lunar House
Globe Park
Marlow
Bucks SL7 1LW
(01628) 488011

Loveridge
J. M. Loveridge plc
Southbrook Road
Southampton
SO15 1BH
(01703) 228411

Loxley
Loxley Medical
Unit 5D, Carnaby
  Industrial Estate
Bridlington
North Humberside
YO15 3QY
(01262) 603979

LRC
LRC Products Ltd
North Circular Road
Chingford
London E4 8QA
0181–527 2377

Lundbeck
Lundbeck Ltd
Sunningdale House
Caldecott Lake
  Business Park
Caldecott
Milton Keynes
MK7 8LF
(01908) 649966

3M
3M Health Care Ltd
3M House
Morley Street

Loughborough
Leics LE11 1EP
(01509) 611611

Maersk
Maersk Medical Ltd
Thornhill Road
North Moons Moat
Redditch
Worcs B98 9NL
(01527) 64222

Manfred Sauer
Manfred Sauer UK
Mill Lane
Eastry
Kent CT13 0QJ
(01304) 620446

Manmed
Mandeville Medicines
Stoke Mandeville
  Hospital
Ayelsbury
Bucks HP21 8AL
(01296) 397223

Marlen
Marlen (UK) Ltd
Unit F4C
Keighley Business
  Centre
South Street
Keighley
West Yorkshire
BD21 1AG
(01535) 610300

Martindale
Martindale
  Pharmaceuticals Ltd
Bampton Road
Harold Hill

Romford
Essex RM3 8UG
(01708) 386660

Medac
Medac GmbH
Fehlandstraße 3
D–2000 Hamburg 36
Germany
(00 49 40) 3509020

Medasil
Medasil (Surgical) Ltd
Medasil House
Hunslet Road
Leeds LS10 1AU
(0113) 243 3491

Medic-Aid
Medic-Aid Ltd
Hook Lane
Pagham
Sussex PO21 3PP
(01243) 267321

Medigas
Medigas Ltd
Enterprise Drive
Four Ashes
Wolverhampton
WV10 7DF
(01902) 791944

Mediplus
Mediplus Ltd
Guildmaster Works
Desborough Road
High Wycombe
Bucks HP11 2QA
(01494) 536222

MediSense
MediSense Britain Ltd

16–17 The Courtyard
Gorsey Lane
Coleshill
Birmingham B46 1JA
(01675) 467044

Medix
Medix Ltd, *see* Clement
  Clarke.

Medo
Medo Pharmaceuticals
  Ltd, *see* Schwarz.

Mepra-pharm
Mepra-pharm
PO Box 4
Rickmansworth
Herts WD3 4AU

Merck
E. Merck
  Pharmaceuticals
Harrier House
High Street
West Drayton
Middx UB7 7QG
(01895) 452200

Merrell
Marion Merrell Dow
  Ltd
Lakeside House
Stockley Park
Uxbridge
Middx UB11 1BE
0181–848 3456

Milupa
Milupa Ltd
Milupa House
Uxbridge Road
Hillingdon

Middx UB10 0NE
0181–573 9966

MMG
MMG (Europe) Ltd
157 Redland Road
Bristol BS6 6YE
(0117) 973 6883

Molnlycke
Molnlycke Ltd
Southfields Road
Dunstable
Beds LU6 3EJ
(01582) 600211

Monmouth
Monmouth
  Pharmaceuticals
3/4 Huxley Road
The Surrey Research
  Park
Guildford
Surrey GU2 5RE
(01483) 65299

Morson
Thomas Morson
  Pharmaceuticals, *see*
  MSD.

MSD
Merck Sharp & Dohme
  Ltd
Hertford Road
Hoddesdon
Herts EN11 9BU
(01992) 467272

Napp
Napp Laboratories Ltd
Cambridge Science
  Park

Milton Road
Cambridge CB4 4GW
(01223) 424444

Nationwide Ostomy
Nationwide Ostomy
  Supplies Ltd
North West House
62 Oakhill Trading
  Estate
Walkden
Manchester M28 5PT
(01204) 709255

Nestlé
Nestlé UK Ltd
St. George's House
Croydon CR9 1NR
0181–686 3333

Network Management
Network Management
  Ltd
Christy Estate
North Lane
Aldershot
Hants GU12 4QP
(01252) 29911

Neutrogena
Neutrogena
  Corporation, *see* J&J

NeXstar
NeXstar
  Pharmaceuticals Ltd
The Quorum
Barnwell Road
Cambridge CB5 8RE
(01223) 571400

Nordic
Nordic Pharmaceuticals
  Ltd, see Ferring.
0181–898 8665

Norgine
Norgine Ltd
Chaplin House
Moorhall Road
Harefield
Middx UB9 6NS
(01895) 826600

Norma
Norma Chemicals Ltd,
  see Wallace Mfg.

North West
North West Medical
  Supplies Ltd
Green Arms Road
Bolton BL7 0ND
(01204) 852383

Norton
H. N. Norton & Co.
  Ltd
Gemini House
Flex Meadow
Harlow
Essex CM19 5TJ
(01279) 426666

Novex
Novex Pharma Ltd
Innovex House
Marlow Park
Marlow
Bucks SL7 1TB
(01628) 491500

Novo Nordisk
Novo Nordisk
  Pharmaceutical Ltd

Novo Nordisk House
Broadfield Park
Brighton Road
Pease Pottage
Crawley
West Sussex RH11 9RT
(01293) 613555

Nutricia Clinical
Nutricia Clinical Care,
  see Cow & Gate

Nutricia Dietary
Nutricia Dietary
  Products Ltd, see Cow
  & Gate

Nycomed
Nycomed (UK) Ltd
Nycomed House
2111 Coventry
Road Sheldon
Birmingham B26 3EA
0121-742 2444

Oakmed
Oakmed Ltd
Fleming Road
Speke
Liverpool L24 9LS
0151-486 3551

Omni Triage
Omni Triage Medical
  Ltd
131 Tranmere Road
London SW18 3QP
0171-737 7781

Omnicare
The Omnicare Group
  Ltd
Enterprise Drive

Four Ashes
Wolverhampton
WV10 7DH
0500 823773

Opus
Opus Pharmaceuticals,
 see Trinity

Oral B Labs
Oral B Laboratories
 Ltd
Gatehouse Road
Aylesbury
Bucks HP19 3ED
(01296) 432601

Organon
Organon Laboratories
 Ltd
Cambridge Science
 Park
Milton Road
Cambridge CB4 4FL
(01223) 423445

Organon-Teknika
Organon-Teknika Ltd,
 see Organon
(01223) 423650

Orion
Orion Pharma (UK)
 Ltd
1st Floor, Leat House
Overbridge Square
Hambridge Lane
Newbury
Berkshire RG14 5UX
(01635) 520300

Orphan Europe
Orphan Europe (UK)

Bray Business Centre
Bray-on-Thames
Berkshire SL6 2ED
(01628) 773342

Ortho
Ortho Pharmaceutical
 Ltd, *see* Cilag.

Orthotic
Orthotic Services Ltd
Heartlands House
19 Catro Street
The Heartlands
Birmingham B7 4TS
0121-359 6323

Owen Mumford
Owen Mumford Ltd
Brook Hill
Woodstock
Oxford OX20 1TU
(01993) 812021

Oxford Nutrition
Oxford Nutrition Ltd
PO Box 110
Witney
Oxon OX8 7FJ
(01993) 709752

**Oxygen Therapy Co
 Ltd**
The Oxygen Therapy
 Co Ltd
Dumballs Road
Cardiff CF1 6JE
0800 373580

Paines & Byrne
Paines & Byrne Ltd
Brocades House
Pyrford Road

West Byfleet
Surrey KT14 6RA
(01932) 355405

Panpharma
Panpharma Ltd
Panpharma House
Repton Place
White Lion Road
Little Chalfont
Amersham
Bucks HP7 9LP
(01494) 766866

Parema
Parema Ltd
Sullington Road
Shepshed
Loughborough
Leics LE12 9JJ
(01509) 502051

Pari
Pari Medical Ltd
London House
243–53 Lower Mortlake
    Road
Richmond
Surrey TW9 2LL
0181-332 6513

Pasteur Mérieux
Pasteur Mérieux MSD
    Ltd
Clivemont House
Clivemont Road
Maidenhead
Berks SL6 7BU
(01628) 785291

Payne
S G & P Payne

Percy House Brook
    Street
Hyde
Cheshire SK14 2NS
0161-367 8561

P-D
Parke-Davis Medical
Lambert Court
Chestnut Avenue
Eastleigh
Hants SO53 3ZQ
(01703) 620500

Pelican
Pelican Healthcare Ltd,
    see Simpla
(01222) 747787

Penn
Penn Pharmaceuticals
    Ltd
Tafarnaubach
    Industrial Estate
Tredegar
Gwent NP2 3AA
(01495) 711222

Pennine
Pennine Healthcare
Pontefract Street
Ascot Drive
Industrial Estate
Derby DE2 8JD
(01332) 384489

Perstorp
Perstorp Pharma Ltd
Wound-Care Division,
    Intec 2
Wade Road
Basingstoke

Hants RG24 8NE
(01256) 477868

Pfizer
Pfizer Ltd
Sandwich
Kent CT13 9NJ
(01304) 616161

Pfizer Consumer
Pfizer Consumer
  Healthcare
Wilsom Road
Alton
Hants GU34 2TJ
(01420) 84801

Pharmacia
see Pharmacia &
  Upjohn

Pharmacia & Upjohn
Pharmacia & Upjohn
  Ltd
Davy Avenue
Knowlhill
Milton Keynes
MK5 8PH
(01908) 661101

Pharmacia-Leiras
Pharmacia-Leiras Ltd,
  see Pharmacia &
  Upjohn.

Pharmark
Pharmark,
7 Windermere Road
West Wickham
Kent BR4 9AN

Pharmax
Pharmax Ltd
Bourne Road

Bexley
Kent DA5 1NX
(01322) 550550

Phillip Harris
Phillip Harris Medical
  Ltd
Hazelwell Lane
Birmingham B30 2PS
0121-433 3030

Phoenix
Phoenix
  Pharmaceuticals Ltd
Glevum Works
Upton Street
Gloucester GL1 4LA
(01452) 522255

Pickles
J. Pickles & Sons
Beech House
62 High Street
Knaresborough
N. Yorks HG5 0EA
(01423) 867314

Portex
Portex Ltd
Hythe
Kent CT21 6JL
(01303) 260551

Procea
Procea
Alexandra Road
Dublin 1.
Dublin 741741

Procter & Gamble
Procter & Gamble
  (Health & Beauty
  Care) Ltd

The Heights
Brooklands
Weybridge
Surrey KT13 0XP
(01932) 896000

**Procter & Gamble
Pharm.**
Procter & Gamble
Pharmaceuticals UK
  Ltd
Lovett House
Lovett Road
Staines
Middx TW18 3AZ
(01784) 495000

Quinoderm Ltd
Quinoderm Ltd
Manchester Road
Hollinwood,
Oldham
Lancs OL8 4PB
0161-624 9307

Rand Rocket
Rand Rocket Ltd
ABCare House
Hownsgill
Industrial Park
Consett
County Durham
DH8 7NU
(01207) 591099

R & C
Reckitt & Colman
  Products Ltd
Dansom Lane
Hull HU8 7DS
(01482) 326151

Regent
Regent Laboratories
  Ltd
Cunard Road
London NW10 6PN
0181-965 3637

Renacare
Renacare Ltd
Nunn Brook Road
Huthwaite
Sutton-in-Ashfield
Notts NG17 2HU
(01623) 555809

Rhône-Poulenc Rorer
Rhône-Poulenc Rorer
  Ltd
52 St. Leonards Road
Eastbourne
East Sussex BN21 3YG
(01323) 534000

Richborough
see Pfizer.

Rima
Rima Pharmaceuticals
  Ltd
214–16 St. James's
  Road
Croydon
Surrey CR0 2BW
0181-683 1266

Robinsons
Robinson Healthcare
Hipper House
Chesterfield
Derbyshire S40 1YF
(01246) 220022

RoC
Laboratories RoC UK
Ltd, *see* J & J

Roche
Roche Products Ltd
PO Box 8
Welwyn Garden City
Herts AL7 3AY
(01707) 366000

**Roche Consumer
Health**
see Roche

Rona
see Lipha

Rosemont
Rosemont
Pharmaceuticals Ltd
Rosemont House
Yorkdale
Industrial Park
Braithwaite Street
Leeds LS11 9XE
(0113) 244 1999

Roussel
see Hoechst Roussel

Rüsch
Rüsch UK Ltd
PO Box 138
Cressex Industrial
Estate
High Wycombe
Bucks HP12 3NB
(01494) 532761

Rybar
Rybar Laboratories Ltd,
see Shire

Sallis
E. Sallis Ltd

Vernon Works
Waterford Street
Basford
Nottingham
NG6 0DH
(0115) 978 7841

Salts
Salt & Son Ltd
Saltair House
Lord Street
Heartlands
Birmingham B7 4DS
0121-359 5123

Sandoz
Sandoz
Pharmaceuticals
Frimley Business Park
Frimley
Camberley
Surrey GU16 5SG
(01276) 692255

Sanofi Winthrop
Sanofi Winthrop Ltd
One Onslow Street
Guildford,
Surrey GU1 4YS
(01483) 505515

Sara Lee
Sara Lee Household &
Personal Care (UK)
Ltd
225 Bath Road
Slough SL1 4AU
(01753) 523971

Schering Health
Schering Health Care
Ltd
The Brow

Burgess Hill
West Sussex RH15 9NE
(01444) 232323

Schering-Plough
Schering-Plough Ltd
Shire Park
Welwyn Garden City
Herts AL7 1TW
(01707) 363636

Scholl
Scholl Consumer
  Products Ltd
475 Capability Green
Luton
Beds LU1 3LU
(01582) 482929

Schwarz
Schwarz Pharma Ltd
Schwarz House
East Street
Chesham
Bucks HP5 1DG
(01494) 772071

**Scientific Hospital
  Supplies**
Scientific Hospital
  Supplies (UK) Ltd
100 Wavertree
  Boulevard
Wavertree Technology
  Park
Liverpool L7 9PT
0151-228 1992

Scotia
Scotia Pharmaceuticals
  Ltd
Units 26–29, Surrey
  Technology Centre

The Research Park
40 Occam Road
Guildford
Surrey GU2 5YG
(01483) 462500

Searle
Searle Pharmaceuticals
PO Box 53
Lane End Road
High Wycombe
Bucks HP12 4HL
(01494) 521124

Serono
Serono Laboratories
  (UK) Ltd
99 Bridge Road East
Welwyn Garden City
Herts AL7 1BG
(01707) 331972

Servier
Servier Laboratories
  Ltd
Fulmer Hall
Windmill Road
Fulmer
Slough SL3 6HH
(01753) 662744

Seton
Seton Healthcare
Seton Healthcare
  Group plc
Tubiton House
Medlock Street
Oldham
Lancs OL1 3HS
0161-652 2222

Seton-Prebbles
see Seton

Seven Seas
Seven Seas Ltd
Hedon Road
Marfleet
Hull HU9 5NJ
(01482) 375234

Seward
Seward Medical
131 Great Suffolk
Street
London SE1 1PP
0171-357 6527

Shannon
T. J. Shannon Ltd
59 Bradford Street
Bolton BL2 1HT
(01204) 21789

Shaw
A. H. Shaw and
Partners Ltd
Manor Road
Ossett
West Yorkshire
WF5 0LF
(01924) 273474

Sherwood
Sherwood Medical
Industries Ltd
County Oak Way
Crawley
West Sussex RH11 7YQ
(01293) 534501

Shire
Shire Pharmaceuticals
Ltd
Fosse House
East Anton Court
Icknield Way

Andover
Hants SP10 5RG
(01264) 333455

Sigma
Sigma Pharmaceuticals
plc
PO Box 233
Watford
Herts WD2 4EW
(01923) 250201

Simcare
Simcare
Peter Road
Lancing
West Sussex BN15 8TJ
(01903) 761122

Simpla
Simpla Plastics Ltd
Cardiff Business Park
Cardiff CF4 5WP
(01222) 747000

Sinclair
Sinclair
Pharmaceuticals Ltd
Borough Road
Godalming
Surrey GU7 2AB
(01483) 426644

S&N Hlth.
Smith & Nephew
Healthcare Ltd
Healthcare House
Goulton Street
Hull HU3 4DJ
(01482) 222200

SK&F
Smith Kline & French
  Laboratories: *see*
  SmithKline Beecham.

SmithKline Beecham
SmithKline Beecham
  Pharmaceuticals
SmithKline Beecham
  plc
Mundells
Welwyn Garden City
Herts AL7 1EY
(01707) 325111

**SmithKline Beecham
  Healthcare**
SmithKline Beecham
Consumer Healthcare
St. Georges Avenue
Weybridge
Surrey KT13 0DE
(01932) 822000

SNBTS
Scottish National Blood
Transfusion Service
Protein Fractionation
  Centre
21 Ellen's Glen Road
Edinburgh EH17 7QT
0131-664 2317

Solvay
Solvay Health Ltd
Hamilton House
Gaters Hill
West End
Southampton
SO18 3JD.
(01703) 472281

Speywood
Speywood
  Pharmaceuticals Ltd
1 Bath Road
Maidenhead
Berks SL6 4UH
(01628) 771417

Squibb
E. R. Squibb & Sons
  Ltd, *see* Bristol-Myers.

Stafford-Miller
Stafford-Miller Ltd
Broadwater Road
Welwyn Garden City
Herts AL7 3SP
(01707) 331001

STD Pharmaceutical
STD Pharmaceutical
  Products
Fields Yard
Plough Lane
Hereford HR4 0EL
(01432) 353684

Steeper
Steeper (Orthopaedic)
  Ltd
Unit 4D, Mead Rise
Temple Gate
Bristol BS3 4RP
(0117) 971 7436

Sterling Health
see SmithKline
  Beecham Healthcare

Sterwin
see Sanofi Winthrop

Stiefel
Stiefel Laboratories
  (UK) Ltd

Holtspur Lane
Wooburn Green
High Wycombe
Bucks HP10 0AU
(01628) 524966

Storz
Storz Ophthalmics
154 Fareham Road
Gosport
Hants PO13 0AS
(01329) 224000

Stuart
see Zeneca

Sussex
Sussex Pharmaceutical
  Ltd
Charlwoods Road
East Grinstead
Sussex RH19 2HL
(01342) 311311

Sutherland
Sutherland Health Ltd
Unit 5, Rivermead
Pipers Way
Thatcham
Berks RG13 4EP
(01635) 874488

Terumo
Terumo Europe N.V.
1st Floor Offices
62 Mount Pleasant
  Road
Tunbridge Wells
Kent TN1 1RB
(01892) 526331

Thackraycare
see DePuy

Thames
see Consolidated

Thornton & Ross
Thornton & Ross Ltd
Linthwaite Laboratories
Huddersfield
HD7 5QH
(01484) 842217

Tillomed
Tillomed Laboratories
  Ltd
Unit 2, Campus 5
Letchworth Business
  Park
Letchworth
Garden City
Herts SG6 2JF
(01462) 480344

Timesco
Timesco of London
Timesco House
1 Knights Road
London E16 2AT
0171-511 1234

Torbet
Torbet Laboratories
  Ltd
Pearl Assurance House
Mill Street
Maidstone
Kent ME15 6XH
(01622) 762269

Tosara
Tosara Products Ltd
Baldoyle Industrial
  Estate
Grange Road

Dublin 13
Dublin 321199

Trinity
Trinity Pharmaceuticals
  Ltd
Tuition House
27-37 St. George's Road
Wimbledon
London SW19 4DS.
0181-944 9443

Typharm
Typharm Ltd
14 Parkstone Road
Poole
Dorset BH15 2PG
(01202) 666626

UCB Pharma
UCB Pharma Ltd
Star House
69 Clarendon Road
Watford
Herts WD1 1DJ
(01923) 211811

Ultrapharm
Ultrapharm Ltd
PO Box 18
Henley-on-Thames
Oxon RG9 2AW
(01491) 578016

Unigreg
Unigreg Ltd
Enterprise House
181–9 Garth Road
Morden
Surrey SM4 4LL
0181-330 1421

Unipath
Unipath Ltd

Norse Road
Bedford MK41 0QG
(01234) 347161

Universal
Universal Hospital
  Supplies
313 Chase Road
London N14 6JA
0181-882 6444

Uno Plast
Uno Plast Ltd
The Wykeham
  Industrial Estate
Moorside Road
Winchester
Hants SO23 7RX.
(01962) 841777

Upjohn
Upjohn Ltd, *see*
  Pharmacia & Upjohn

Vernon-Carus
Vernon-Carus Ltd
Penwortham Mills
Preston
Lancs PR1 9SN
(01772) 744493

Vestric
Vestric Ltd
West Lane
Runcorn
Cheshire WA7 2PE
(01928) 717070

Vitabiotics
Vitabiotics Ltd
Vitabiotics House
3 Bashley Road
London NW10 6SU
0181-963 0999

Vitaflo
Vitaflo Ltd
6 Moss Street
Paisley PA1 1BJ
0800 515174

Vitalograph
Vitalograph Ltd
Maids Moreton House
Maids Moreton
Buckingham
MK18 1SW
(01280) 822811

Vygon
Vygon (UK) Ltd
Bridge Road
Cirencester
Glos GL7 1PT
(01285) 657051

H. G. Wallace
H. G. Wallace Ltd
Colchester
Essex CO2 8JH
(01206) 795133

Wallace Mfg
Wallace Manufacturing
Chemists Ltd
Randles Road
Knowsley Industrial
  Park
Merseyside L34 9HX
0151-549 1255

Wanskerne
Wanskerne Ltd
31 High Cross Street
St. Austell

Cornwall PL25 4AN
(01726) 69500

Ward
Ward Surgical
  Appliance Co Ltd
57A Brightwell Avenue
Westcliffe-on-Sea
Essex SS0 9EB
(01702) 354064

Warner Wellcome
Warner Wellcome
  Consumer
  Healthcare, *see* P-D

WBP
WB Pharmaceuticals
  Ltd, *see* Boehringer
  Ingelheim

Welfare Foods
see Nutricia

Welland
Welland Medical Ltd
7 Brunel Centre
Newton Road
Crawley
West Sussex RH10 2TU
(01293) 615455

Wellcome
see Glaxo Wellcome

Whitehall
Whitehall Laboratories
  Ltd
Huntercombe Lane
  South
Taplow
Maidenhead

Berks SL6 0PH
(01628) 669011

Willis
S. R. Willis & Sons Ltd
176 Albion Road
London N16 9JR
0171-254 7373

Windsor
see Boehringer
 Ingelheim

W-L
Warner Lambert UK
 Ltd, *see* P-D

Wyeth
Wyeth Laboratories
Huntercombe Lane
 South
Taplow
Maidenhead
Berks SL6 0PH
(01628) 604377

Wyvern
Wyvern Medical Ltd
PO Box 17
Ledbury
Herefordshire HR8 2ES
(01531) 631105

Yamanouchi
Yamanouchi Pharma
 Ltd
Yamanouchi House
Pyrford Road
West Byfleet
Surrey KT14 6RA
(01932) 345535

Zeal
G. H. Zeal Ltd
8 Lombard Road
Merton
London SW19 3UU.
0181-542 2283

Zeneca
Zeneca Pharma
King's Court
Water Lane
Wilmslow
Cheshire SK9 5AZ
(01625) 712712

Zyma
Zyma Healthcare
Mill Road
Holmwood
Dorking
Surrey RH5 4NU
(01306) 742800

'Special-order' manufacturers
The following *companies* manufacture 'special-order' products: BCM Specials, Martindale, Rosemont *Hospital manufacturing units* also manufacture 'special-order' products, details may be obtained from any of the centres listed below. It should be noted that when a product has a licence the Department of Health recommends that the licensed product should be ordered unless a specific formulation is required.

England

East Anglian and Oxford

Mr G. Hanson
Regional Production
   Pharmacist
Pharmacy Department
The Ipswich Hospital
Heath Road
Ipswich
Suffolk IP4 5PD
(01473) 712233 Extn
   5603

Mersey

Dr M. G. Lee
Regional Quality
   Control Pharmacist
Pharmacy Practice Unit
70 Pembroke Place
Liverpool L69 3BX
0151–794 8138

North Thames

Mr M. Lillywhite
Regional Production
   Pharmacist
St. Bartholomew's
   Hospital
West Smithfield
London EC1A 7BE
0171–601 7477

North Western

Mr M. D. Booth
Production & Aseptic
   Services Manager
Stockport
   Pharmaceuticals
Stepping Hill Hospital
Stockport

Cheshire SK2 7JE
0161–419 5657

Northern

Mr P. W. McKenzie
Regional Technical
   Services Pharmacist
Pharmacy Department
Newcastle General
   Hospital
Westgate Road
Newcastle upon Tyne
NE4 6BE
0191–273 8811 Extn
   22479

South East Thames

Mr J. Cheetham
Principal Pharmacist
Guy's Hospital
St. Thomas' Street
London SE1 9RT
0171–955 5000 Extn
   5378/3712

South West Thames

Mr S. J. Riley
Regional Production
   Pharmacist
Pharmacy Department
Lanesborough Wing
St. George's Hospital
Blackshaw Road
Tooting
London SW17 0QT
0181–725 1770

Southern Western

Mr C. W. Lewis
Director
Manorpark
   Pharmaceuticals

Blackberry Hill
   Hospital
Manor Road
Bristol BS16 2EW
(0117) 975 4852

Trent
Mr A. C. Moore
Regional Production
   Representative
Royal Hallamshire
   Hospital
Glossop Road
Sheffield S10 2JF
(0114) 271 2325

Wessex
Dr E. Brierley
Regional
   Manufacturing Unit
Queen Alexandra
   Hospital
Cosham
Portsmouth
Hants PO6 3LY
(01705) 286335

West Midlands
Mr P. G. Williams
Principal Pharmacist
Pharmacy
   Manufacturing Unit
Burton Hospital NHS
   Trust
Belvedere Road
Burton-on-Trent
DE13 0RB
(01283) 566333 Extn
   5138

Yorkshire
Mr E. Holt

Principal Pharmacist
Production Unit
The Royal Infirmary
Acre Street
Lindley
Huddersfield
West Yorks HD3 3EA
(01484) 422191 Extn
   2421

Northern Ireland
Mrs S. M. Millership
Principal Pharmacist
Central Pharmaceutical
   Production Unit
CSA Distribution
   Centre
77 Boucher Crescent
Belfast BT12 6HU
(01232) 553407

Scotland
Mr J. A. Cook
Principal Pharmacist –
   Regional Production
Tayside
   Pharmaceuticals
Ninewells Hospital
Dundee DD1 9SY
(01382) 632273

Wales
Mr C. Powell
Specialist Principal
   Pharmacist
Sterile Products Unit
Pharmacy Department
University Hospital of
   Wales

The Heath
Cardiff CF4 4XW

(01222) 747747 Extn
3114

USEFUL TELEPHONE AND BLEEP NUMBERS

Consultant _____

Consultant _____

Consultant _____

Consultant _____

Consultant _____

Consultant _____

Senior Registrar _____

Registrar _____

SHO _____

Anaesthetist _____

Accident & Emergency _____

Administrator _____

Biochemistry _____

Cardiology _____

Chest Physician _____

Community Psychiatric Nurse _____

Cytology _____

Dermatology _____

ECT _____

Gastroenterology _____

Haematology _____

Immunology _____

Microbiology _____

Neurology _____

Nursing Officer _____

Occupational Health _____

Occupational Therapy _____

Pathology _____

Pharmacy _____

Porters _____

Psychology _____

Psychotherapy _____

Renal medicine _____

Social Worker _____

Virology _____

X-ray _____

Wards _____

_____

_____

_____

Secretary _____

Medical Records _____

_____

_____

_____

_____

_____

_____

INDEX